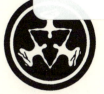

MENOPAUSE & BEYOND

A Fitness Plan For Life

By

Leora Myers, R.N.

Adelaide Press
San Francisco, California

ISBN 0-9647666-0-4
First Edition 1995
Printed in the United States of America

Project Manager/Editor: Laura Kath
Book Design & Typesetting: Peggy Ferris
Mariah Marketing; Santa Barbara, California

In view of the complex, individual and specific
nature of health and fitness problems, this book is not
intended to replace professional medical advice.
The author/publisher expressly disclaim responsibility for any liability, loss or risk, personal or other-
wise, which is incurred as a consequence, directly or
indirectly, from the use and application of any of the
contents of this book.

Front Cover Photo:
"This is what fifty looks like!"
-Leora Myers, R.N.

THIS BOOK IS DEDICATED TO:

Adelaide, Leora and Marie

My Mother and Grandmothers, who taught me strength
and wisdom.

Lyman

My Father, who inspired my tenacity.

Dennis

My Husband, whose patience, love and understanding
was the encouragement to "do it".

Michael

My Son, my creative inspiration.

*Lyman Jr., Georgianna, Ethel,
Lutzie and Adelaide*

My Brother and Sisters, whose challenges made me
earn the title of being "Big Sis".

Acknowledgments

"Leora, it's time to give birth to this baby," my editor Laura Kath's words illustrated the truth of the moment, pointedly referring to the fact that I had carried this manuscript around with me for almost nine months and felt ready to burst, to scream, to cry out. My moment, my decision to self-publish this "baby" in April 1995, manifested like a birth of an overdue pregnancy, and eventually came complete with Lamaze classes filled with true friends supporting, encouraging and deep breathing with me all the way.

First, I would like to thank Carolyn Cogan, Aerobics Director, Jewish Community Center, San Rafael, California, for selecting me to be her keynote speaker, as well as respecting and giving value to my decision to speak publicly for the first time about menopause.

Thanks to Evelyn White, editor, *Black Women's Health Book* (Seal Press), for inviting me to contribute to the updated version by writing the chapter, "New Frontiers: Black Women and Menopause," my first published work; and especially for telling me that I am a writer.

I thank all the women who came to my workshops on menopause and openly shared their experiences; as well as giving value and appreciation for the information they received, and asked questions requiring me to continue the study of menopause.

For Dr. Sadja Greenwood, my mentor and inspiration, for encouraging me to write this book on fitness for women going through menopause.

To Berit Muh, who patiently helped me understand how a computer works and how not to lose my manuscript.

For Christy Wright, who, at the last moment, came through with a transcript of my workshop, and Martha Kirsten, who assisted in the process.

To Ann Bullwinkel and Irene Teglia McKay for your encouragement and kind acts of support.

To Paul Hupf, your legal (and life) advice has always encouraged me to excel in every endeavor.

To all the women of the first "Mid-life & Beyond Support Group"--as well as Jim and Linda Gerber, Sandy Minor and Bruce Valentine of Western

Athletic Clubs, that supported the vision by providing meeting space for our groups at Pacific Athletic Club, Redwood City, California.

To Linda Krassner, your strength and humor moved me to continue.

To Rich Baker, your advice between sets was invaluable.

To Fumiko Makiba, your encouragement gave me that "don't give up" spirit and helped me realize the seasons of my life.

To all my students at the Leora Myers & Co. Fitness Center, Donnelly Square, Pacific Athletic Club, Telegraph Hill Club and the Weight Management Program. You are my inspiration!

To Leon Pleasant, my personal trainer who patiently listened to my "hot flash" complaints between sets and then proceeded to give the usual tough workout, as always!

To Pamela Price Lechtman, my very own fairy godmother! Thank you again for moving me along in life's endeavors with your introduction to my editor, Laura Kath. Your words, "you've got to write this book" kept me at the computer through the nights.

To Rhodessa Jones, you transform women's lives with your honesty. Thank you for inviting me to be part of your vision.

To Maya Lit, thank you for sharing your remarkable talent to choose the colors, textures and design that make for "more than just a wardrobe."

My most sincere gratitude to Sensei!

And finally, to the two Leos that roared . . . Laura Kath, Project Manager/ Editor and Peggy Ferris, Graphic Designer . . . you are ladies of my heart with vision, determination and a "kick butt" attitude that I needed. THANK YOU!!!!!

Credits
✤

Photography: Kevin Bond
Cover photo hair : Margo Tomasini
Make-up: Lisa Jear

Table of Contents

Foreword

This book is a huge and important undertaking. We all have questions about menopause and beyond. No one has all the answers. Perhaps the best approach is a process of gaining understanding of our own bodies as they change, inside and out, and being willing to make the commitment to nurture the best in each of us.

Leora first came into my life when my office manager proposed that our staff exercise together. My initial thought was, "This will blow over pretty fast." But she said she had found a truly extraordinary trainer, and I was intrigued.

When I put on my tights and leotard and showed up at the Leora Myers Fitness Center studio, I realized that she was the lady with the intimidating body, whose announcements about "The Best Workout in Town" I had seen–and avoided– many times. My original doubts soon changed to commitment, as I felt increased strength, balance and pleasure, both physically and emotionally, resulting from this work. We, as a staff, soon began to eagerly anticipate the challenge and rewards of our workouts together. When we moved to a new location, we planned our own fitness room with mirrors and a sound system, especially for our classes with Leora.

Leora's message and methods stem from a truly special blend of medical knowledge, training, experience, insight, compassion, tenacity and humor. It is now nine years later, and Leora, with her class, and fitness classes, are still an integral part of my personal and professional life. Leora's lifestyle and attitudes about healthfulness in all realms have touched us deeply. We have seen her adapt to the agenda that her life plays out, sometimes philosophical and patient, sometimes skeptical and feisty, but always with consideration and integrity. As for me, I entered menopause, developed a lung disease that required years of high-dose steroids, had shoulder surgery, and my share of emotional pains and pleasures.

Through it all, Leora has provided that persistent, gentle pressure to be my physical and mental best.

I know that you, too, will learn from Leora, and that this book will contribute importantly to your own life process. To your health, through menopause and beyond!

Joan Saxton, M.D.
Fellow, American College of Physicians
San Francisco, California

Introduction

"We must never forget that we may also find meaning in life when confronted with a hopeless situation, when facing a fate that cannot be changed. When we are no longer able to change a situation—we are challenged to change ourselves."

VICTOR FRANKEL

Warming Up

A Personal Note About the "Change"

M enopause. This is the term our society uses to collectively describe a woman's passage into a natural but mysterious aspect of life. In the past, many women have avoided even thinking about "it," until they have that first hot flash; then, make a fast dash to the physician for a hormone prescription for "immediate relief."

Today, as we see "baby boomer" women approaching the Big M, we see a new urgency to know what to expect, and to better prepare for this event. We are no longer willing to sweat in silence, or lie down and suffer silently. Unlike our mothers and grandmothers, who so often would escape to the back porch to fan that hot flash away, we are completely involved in living our life to the fullest–running companies, leading board meetings, completing major projects, raising families, protecting our environment and preserving our communities. When that dreaded flash appears, we fully realize that the fan and a back porch are not handy, and besides, we just don't have time for such nuisances.

The controversial decision of hormone replacement therapy (HRT) treatment will be a volatile issue for women and will rival the pro-choice issue of today when forty million American women will have begun "the change" by the year 2020– certainly a clear description of global warming!

My personal passage through menopause has been shocking, depressing, encouraging and humorous; sometimes all at once! After experiencing that first hot flash, I knew I wanted to know more about this stage in my life. I have found it surprisingly hopeful and interesting. I am inspired by the opportunities in my horizon to make this a powerful time of life. My flashes came after several months of irregular periods. My first warning came as I noticed that the day after my weekly hair appointment, my hair was a mess! I always was envied by my friends as the one with the beautiful hair– that looked great even days after my appointment. I complained to my hairdresser, of course. She gave me "The Look" (which I later came to understand as–you must be going through "The Change") and she admitted, "Well, your hair may be going through some changes . . . that does happen."

My second clue came when I was teaching one of my daily fitness classes. I felt very warm and shouted, "Is it hot in here or is it just me?" One of my "mature" clients winked and gave me "The Look." The real cooker (every pun intended) occurred when I, who could sleep through a four alarm fire, began waking up two or three times a night, just perspiring like crazy. Still, I was not getting the hint that I was experiencing night sweats. I always had liked to sleep toasty warm, wrapped in an electric blanket on my side of the bed, since my husband Dennis hates heat and likes to sleep cool with a nearby window wide open.

One night, my husband rolled over and sternly said, "Turn off that blanket!"
I immediately sobbed, "The blanket isn't on!"
At that moment, reality finally came crashing in, and I knew that my body was going through The Change.

At first I protested to anyone I thought might care (family, friends and students alike will testify) "I am not going to go through this!" Of course, this cry was as useless as a young girl denying her first menstrual period. I personally tried Hormone Replacement Therapy (HRT), which alleviated my hot flashes almost immediately. However, I encountered other HRT effects including weight gain, awful PMS symptoms and heavy monthly bleeding, which I judged to be just too uncomfortable for me.

Frustrated and feeling hopeless about my physical changes, I sought spiritual guidance through my Buddhist practice. I had a meeting with a trusted advisor who reminded me that "Life is like the seasons and you are in the Autumn of your life. It is also like day and night. It is very natural. We do not argue with the change in the seasons or the change in the day. We accept it and do what is natural at that time of the year or the day. You can make this time of change in your life your friend or your enemy. It is your choice."

I will freely admit that this message was the turning point in my change process. I believe that every woman will have such a moment as she goes through this stage of life. The change agent may be a person, an event or circumstance; perhaps, even reading this book. It is my wish that every woman recognize that menopause and beyond can, if we choose, be a positive life change.

Opportunity Knocks

"In the middle of difficulty lies opportunity"
-Albert Einstein

Dateline: May 3, 1993
San Rafael, California
2nd Annual Fit 'n Fun Day for Women Over 40

The event organizer's words blaze into the enthusiastic crowd of 200 women, "This has truly been a great day! Now I wish to introduce our keynote speaker, Leora Myers, sharing her message entitled Mid-life and Menopause: Shedding the Fears, Embracing the Challenge . . ."

As I stood backstage, with my eyes closed, I went through my ritual of deep breathing and a mind game where I list every job I would rather have than the one before me–a waitress, a grocery clerk, a gas station attendant–anything that will save me from the dreaded first few minutes of my speech. I remind myself that once I begin, everything is always okay.

Through my ritual, I hear the introduction and an unexpected shock runs through my body. Did I hear her correctly? I'm giving a talk on MENOPAUSE today? This can't be right! Leora, you have gone crazy! (One of those reported menopausal symptoms!) My carefully prepared speech, what had been intended to be a heroic endeavor–one that saves all womanhood from the dreaded sufferings of The Change– one that would make me the Betty Friedan of Menopause– now seems like one of the dumbest opportunities I've ever considered!

Nonetheless, I walk onto the stage, look out at a room full of women, who all look about as excited as I feel about this "Menopause" topic after a great day of fun and activity. I had already instructed my staff to place packages of M&M's® candies into each guest's information packet–no doubt increasing the skepticism that I was experiencing. Essentially, these women were very confused. This was supposed to be a fitness day–Leora Myers is a nurse, yet she gives us M&M's® in her materials? "Are we even allowed to eat them here?," someone whispered.

Right then, my strongest urge was to admit to one and all that my very first ever "Menopause" speech was a stupid idea–perhaps we should end this event early, and go enjoy this gorgeous, sunny California day. The podium, always a speaker's security blanket, today is a fragile music stand which barely holds my M&M's® speech notes. Whew! NOTES! I'm so glad I have them, because within the last 20 seconds (that seemed like 20 minutes) my mind has gone completely blank (another reported menopausal symptom, memory loss). Ah ha, that's what I will use as my opening, I think. I forge ahead with these lines.

"Mid-life and menopause. At this time, many women experience short-term memory loss. I know because I have just forgotten the opening to my speech!" The rational part of my brain realizes this is way too flippant and a rather self-depreciating start. I lift my chin, straighten my body, take a deep breath and tell myself, "Leora, this speech IS what you want to do. This is the opportunity you have been waiting for to go public with your research. Let's get on with it!" My mouth opens and out comes the following confident roar!

"Mid-life. Menopause. Two words–for many women, difficult to think about, much less even to say out loud. Today, we will discuss the physical, emotional and spiritual challenges we experience at this time in the journey of our lives. I want you to recognize the myths and be given a clue that like the M&M's® in your packet, there really is a sweetness to this time of life! " An audible chuckle runs through the crowd, there is a reason behind those M&M's® candies after all! It is the same reason I decided to write and publish this book. One year after my first hot flash, I knew that even as a nurse, a fitness trainer, and a practicing health professional, there must be something beyond just the physical symptoms of "The Change" something more than "feeling crazy" emotionally and questioning my spiritual nature. I have researched, studied, meditated, practiced and even cried so much about my menopause over the ensuing years–and I am here to tell you that I have found that sweetness. I feel a compelling need to share this information of my self-study with other women. Information that gives strategy, education and purpose to this natural transition.

This book represents my journey of going through and beyond the passage commonly called menopause; and developing a health and fitness-based guide to the lifestyle choices that can have dramatic beneficial effects on your life . . . today and tomorrow.

What Is Menopause?

Menopause is a permanent ending of menstruation. It literally means the last menstrual period. Menopause represents a change from the reproductive to the nonreproductive years of a woman's life. It is one of the occurrences in the *climacteric*, a biological change happening in women between the ages of forty-five and sixty years. Climacteric is the time when the ovaries stop producing estrogen and a woman's child bearing capability ends.

As you approach your forties, your ovaries are programmed to naturally begin to run out of eggs. The pituitary and hypothalamus glands in the brain control your ovaries. Concurrently, the estrogen that ovaries produce decreases and ovulation becomes irregular. As estrogen decreases, there is a short circuit-like interaction between the signals of the brain for ovulation to begin due to the decreased estrogen. Hence, menopause. The term perimenopause refers to the years leading up to the last menstrual period. Postmenopause pertains to the time after the end of the monthly menarche (monthly menstrual cycle).

All women have different physical and emotional experiences during this time of life. However, research shows that there is a predictable time sequence of symptoms and occurrences to indicate when you are approaching or dealing with menopause on a daily basis.

The following is a sequential look at menopause based on a woman at age fifty:

```
Age: 45-50.....Irregular, heavy or spotty menstrual periods
        48........Hot Flashes
        50........Menopause (technically, the last period)
        52........Hot Flashes
        54........Vaginal Dryness
        56........Bladder Control Loss
        58........Cardiovascular Disease Risk
        60........Osteoporosis Onset
```

Remember, EVERY WOMAN IS DIFFERENT. You or your best friend may just stop having those periods and have no further problems. Other women experience symptoms that cause discomfort ranging from mild to severe.

Since the average age of menopause is fifty-one, but the onset can occur between forty-five and fifty-five, premature menopause is defined as symptoms occurring prior to age forty-five. Some factors attributed to causing menopause to arrive early are:

-Surgical removal of ovaries.
-Infections that destroy ovarian tissue.
-Irradiation or chemotherapy for cancer.
-Smoking more than a half pack of cigarettes a day.
-Heavy alcohol consumption.
-High altitude or elevation.
-Extreme thinness (less than 15% body fat).

Note: The body's fat tissue is capable of converting androgens, produced by the ovaries and adrenal glands, into estrogen. Obese women tend to go through menopause later due to the storage and retention of these androgens. However, this is not to be used as an excuse to be overweight. Obesity risk factors far surpass estrogen deprivation and earlier menopause.

Surgical menopause is when the ovaries are removed, a bilateral oophorectomy along with a hysterectomy, or for medical reasons such as severe endometriosis, pelvic infection or ovarian cysts and tumors. Menopausal symptoms such as hot flashes and night sweats occur within days of surgery and estrogen replacement therapy is usually begun immediately after surgery. A hysterectomy is the surgical removal of the uterus and not the ovaries. This alone should not cause menopausal symptoms except cessation of menstrual cycles. Irregular heavy bleeding can occur with the decrease in ovulation and hormonal output. Many factors such as cigarette smoking, stress and excessive alcohol can worsen this condition, but medical problems such as fibroid tumors may be the cause. Any persistent, abnormal bleeding should be discussed with your physician.

Some Thoughts About Hormone Replacement Therapy (HRT)

I am well aware of the serious question every woman faces at this time of life–Is hormone replacement therapy for me? The guidelines in this book for lifestyle and fitness choices are not intended as a substitute for hormone replacement therapy. That is a decision you personally have to make, along with your physician and healthcare team. Hopefully, I will give you knowledge to make a better-informed decision. However, research indicates that falling estrogen levels are not the only cause for osteoporosis, heart disease, and the weight gains and shifts commonly associated with menopause. Remember, no amount of estrogen (no matter what the source) will protect you from these diseases and symptoms if you have unhealthy lifestyle habits. So after those hot flashes end, what are you going to do with the rest of your life? The second half of your life is a time for health, personal fulfillment and an increased zest for life.

Frankly, I must admit that the "HRT Controversy" has had some revolutionary positive results–a new coming-together of women to discuss menopause more openly and honestly than ever before. This concern of the newly approaching "baby boomers" toward HRT has created other options and healthier attitudes.

The great debate that always brings my "Mid-life & Menopause" workshops to a heated halt sounds something like this. If these concerns are yours, please know that you are not alone! "What will happen if years from now we discover they are harmful? I don't want to be someone's guinea pig. I refuse to take hormones that are manufactured from horses' urine. I am concerned about animal abuse. But, I feel wonderful since I've been taking them. I'm afraid of breast cancer. I refuse to go to a doctor and automatically be put on HRT. I'd rather die at sixty-five of heart disease than fifty-five of breast cancer. I'm so confused. My mood swings and hot flashes vanished. Vaginal dryness was the reason I went on them. I'm afraid not to take my hormones. I know there are some good reasons to take them but . . ."

I am emphatic that my work is not about HRT. I am not willing to advise you one way or another. I made my choice. I have to live with it and all the consequences, and so will you. Study the risk factors for heart disease, breast cancer and osteoporosis carefully. Seek a medical practitioner you trust and one that listens to you–is sensitive to your questions, your thoughts, your concerns. If you take HRT, be willing to find the ideal dosage based on how you feel. BE the collaborator in this process. Come to your medical exam prepared with your questions. Insist on answers and know that your expert medical collaborator is out there if you are not presently satisfied.

My best advice is to plan your lifestyle and fitness choices that include options you have control over–like exercise, diet and relaxation. This book is intended to give you information about improving your quality of life. Even though you may go on hormone replacement therapy and the hot flashes end . . . then what are you going to do with the rest of your life?

What Is Physical Fitness?

A definition: enhanced physiological or functional capacity that allows for an improved quality of life. "Functional fitness" means the physical capacity to meet ordinary and unexpected demands of daily life safely and effectively. It promotes function, physical independence and contributes to an improved health status and reduction of health-related illnesses. Functional fitness (as opposed to traditional physical fitness) is now the recognized definition for fitness in the 90's–the quality of life, or ability to DO life. In other words, physical fitness enables one to function–to do all that life requires with a high level of energy and an overall positive feeling of enthusiasm. A high level of fitness (what you can experience after implementing this plans described in this book) is reflected by physiological adaptations such as lower heart rate and improved ability to utilize body fuels.

The following five components of physical fitness: muscular strength, muscular endurance, cardiovascular/cardiorespiratory capacity, flexibility and body composition, are of equal importance and should be included in every well-rounded program.

l. Increase Muscular Strength
Definition: The force that a muscle can exert during contraction.
To build maximal strength, the load is high and the repetitions are low.
Frequency: Train 2-3 times per week minimum. Rest 24-48 hours for recovery of stress.
Duration: Use weight able to handle no less than 8 repetitions and no more than l2.
Sets: Perform minimum l set per major muscle group. 8-10 exercises.
Technique: Controlled, deliberate movement: 2 count up, pause, 4 count down. Full range of motion.
Sequence: Large to small muscles.
Progress: Increase weight by 5% after 12 reps. Strength gains continue with progressive overload.
Rest: 2-3 minutes to for muscle recovery for maximal lifts.
Equipment: Free weights, machines; props including rubberized resistive tubing and bands, weighted bars and balls.

2. Increase Muscular Endurance
Definition: The number of times a muscle or muscle group can repeatedly exert force against a resistance without fatiguing. Moderate resistance.
To build endurance the load is low and the repetitions are high.

Frequency: 2-3 days per week.
Duration: 12-15 repetitions.
Progress: Achieve 15-20 repetitions maximum.
Rest: 30 seconds between sets.
Equipment: Weights, body weight (calisthenics), use of props such as rubberized resistive tubing, bands and weighted balls.

3. Improve Cardiovascular/Cardiorespiratory Aerobic Fitness

Definition: The capacity of the heart-lung system to deliver blood and oxygen to the working muscles during sustained exercise.
Exercise intensity: 50-85 % of maximum heart rate.
Duration: 20-60 minutes continuous aerobic activity.
Frequency: 3-5 times a week.
Progression: Increase systematically intensity, duration and frequency 5-10% per 2 weeks.
Type: Any activity that uses large muscle groups.
Activities: Walking, running, cycling, swimming, dance exercise, stair climbing, cross country skiing or rowing.
It is important to note that all benefits of cardiovascular and strength training are reversible. Four-six weeks after training there can be almost complete loss of aerobic and strength benefit.

4. Increase Flexibility

Definition: The range of motion possible around a joint over which a muscle or muscle group spans.
Type: Static non-ballistic (bouncing) stretches.
Duration: Held 5-30 seconds.
Progression: Increase range of motion (ROM) to point of tension, not pain.
Frequency: Stretching exercises 5-7 minutes before and after exercise. For enhanced benefit 2 days a week, 15-20 minutes each session.

5. Improve Body Composition

The reduction of body fat is altered by rules of caloric balance–intake vs. expenditure, meal distribution and food source of calories. Lean body mass and basal metabolic rate affects caloric expenditure.

The Benefits of a Fitness Plan For Life

Why am I sold on sharing with you my "Fitness Plan for Life"? I have come to understand, through my personal experiences and those of my students and clients, that higher levels of physical fitness at this important time of life can do the following:

* Increase energy and stamina.
* Improve the nervous system and digestive tract functions.
* Help prevent heart disease.
* Help relieve anxiety, insomnia and depression.
* Control weight.
* Increase body tone.
* Improve muscle strength.
* Gain flexibility and joint range of motion (ROM).
* Help relieve hot flashes.
* Increase bladder control.
* Help relieve vaginal changes.
* Help to prevent osteoporosis and related falls.
* Build strong bones.

This book is dedicated to educating and inspiring you–today's active woman–to take an active and creative role in expanding your horizons–physically, mentally and spiritually.

PART ONE

The Physical Issues

"The events in our lives happen in a sequence in time, but in their significance to ourselves, they find their own order . . . the continuous thread of revelation."

EUDORA WELTY

CHAPTER ONE

Hot Flashes

Dateline: July 1992
Myers Family Reunion
Indianapolis, Indiana

Warm summer nights, endless hide and seek, home cooking to "put some meat on those skinny bones," vacation-time boyfriends, girl talk, sharing dreams of when we get married to "the one," stories of how granddaddy Lyman Myers had married Leora Brown and raised a family of ten–these are all memories of my annual summer vacation in Indianapolis with my cousins, aunts and uncles.

Since I was raised in the north country of Minneapolis/St. Paul, the midwestern style of Indianapolis seemed like a foreign country to me in so many ways. Instead of Sunday Mass, there was the Baptist church service where the songs made me want to dance, followed by Sunday dinner, a feast that my aunts all swore would make me look "much better" when I returned home to Minnesota.

I was always insulted when I was referred to as skinny by my elder relations, but then, I was being compared to the fullness of body shared by most Myers women. We young ones swore we never would let that fate happen to us.

"Yes, she's one of the Myers cousins from up north, that eldest daughter of Lyman. You remember, he was the only son to leave Indianapolis. Went up to St. Paul, Minnesota, to live in the home town of his wife, Adelaide," was the usual way

I was introduced around during those endless summers. It was funny how "Myers" came out sounding like "Marsch" with the southern accent of Indianapolis, but one I easily acquired and proudly kept until returning northward again.

Some thirty years later, when I returned to Indianapolis for our first Myers family reunion, I have married "the one" and have a twenty-seven year old son. I am so excited about seeing my relatives and having meaningful conversations with my cousins about the life we lead today. Cousin Pat meets me at the airport and the first words out of her mouth are, "Leora, are you having hot flashes yet?"

Defining The "Hot Flash"

Hot flashes are the most common complaint of women in menopause and are experienced by seventy-five percent of all women. Hot flashes, also referred to as hot flushes, are characterized by a sudden onset of heat and sweating. The skin temperature goes up approximately four degrees. As perspiring begins to cool the skin, shivering may follow. When they happen at night, they are referred to as "night sweats." You can get the picture of someone pulling off clothes (or sheets), becoming cool and then adding clothing back again; all in the space of two to twenty minutes. Hot flashes may last a few seconds to a few minutes and their characteristics and intensity may change as they come and go over the months. The number of flashes can vary from three a month to over forty a day. Hot flashes do change in characteristics and intensity over time and are dependent upon our particular menopausal clock. Since all of our experiences of menopause are different, fifteen percent of the female population report having very few hot flashes or none at all. "What's the big deal? I think I had one hot flash!" Betty Friedan exclaimed at the 1994 Women of Vision Conference, Washington, DC.

When I began to have hot flashes they were like a flood of heat from my waist to the top of my head; lasted at least a minute and required me to stop whatever I was doing at the time. Today, they are like a summer rainfall over my face and neck, last 15-20 seconds and get my attention only in a passing thought–oh, how interesting, I'm having a hot flash!

What causes hot flashes? Research scientists believe that as the level of estrogen production decreases, there is a change in the brain's chemistry that affects the temperature control center in the hypothalamus, the brain's master gland regulating body temperature–your body thermostat. At menopause, this thermostat incorrectly senses that you are cold and raises your body temperature. The body immediately dilates the blood vessels to cool itself down, you perspire–and have a hot flash. The natural reduction of estrogen within our ovaries during menopause is the recognized factor for the hot flash experience. However, every woman has an individual response to that factor–including varying degrees of frequency, intensity, duration and ultimately, overall discomfort.

Women have vividly described their personal "hot flash" experiences in my Mid-life & Menopause workshops. Each one is different; from its length of time, part of body involved, emotional expression of attitude of the experience. "I've been cold all my life. Hot flashes give me an exhilarating warmth which I enjoy!" "I hate the uncertainty of when I'll get one. I'm embarrassed to turn red and break out in a sweat in public." "I was prepared for the hot flash I knew would have while I was with this other person, so I rehearsed my response. So when I flashed while speaking with a young female employee who said, alarmed "You are so red, are you mad at me?", I confidently said, "No, dear I AM JUST HAVING A HOT FLASH!" "I feel like I'm getting the flu. My joints ache and I am nauseous." "They begin in my face, radiate to the top of my head."

Many women continue producing estrogen from other sources and may have reduced hot flashes. Surgical menopause causes sudden cessation of estrogen production and

immediate hot flashes compared to the gradual estrogen reduction experienced during a traditional menopause. Hot
flashes are usually the first indication of the onset of menopause; and what causes most women to seek relief through
hormone replacement therapy (HRT). Estrogen is not the only
hormone involved in triggering a hot flash. Several other hormones are involved.

What can you do to minimize the hot flash experience? Here
are some lifestyle and fitness choice tips.

LIFESTYLE OPTIONS

Lifestyle choices can lessen the intensity and frequency of
hot flashes. First and foremost, get to know your personal
"flashing pattern" by keeping a daily journal. Write down
these factors about each and every flash for at least one week:

1. When
2. Duration
3. Intensity
4. Situation

You will be able to definitely observe a pattern and more
completely understand what things trigger your hot flashes.
Here are some possible "hot flash" triggers and solutions.

Alcohol
It dilates blood vessels and makes you warmer. Reduce night
sweats by avoiding alcohol consumption at least four hours
before going to bed.

Caffeine
Reduce all foods that contain caffeine. The biggest culprits
are chocolate, coffee, tea and cola. You can significantly reduce night-time flushes by avoiding caffeine after Noon.

Hot, spicy foods
Raise your body temperature in general. Why intensify the effect by consuming more?

Large meals
Try to eat smaller portions, more frequently.

Sugar
Decrease sugar intake since both simple and complex sugars can cause metabolic and mood swings.

Hot, stuffy temperatures in room or environment
Always sleep in a cool, well-ventilated room. Keep cool water at bedside. To get back to sleep after a night sweat, take a warm (not hot) bath and have a complex carbohydrate snack like a banana, some yogurt or whole grain cereal.

Clothing
Wear light cotton clothes that allow your skin and pores to breathe. Avoid polyester and synthetic fabrics since they can trap perspiration. Dress in layers to accommodate a flash. Carry a decorative fan and start a fashion trend.

Water
Make sure you consciously hydrate your body. Drink plenty of cool water throughout the day. The old axiom of eight, eight ounce glasses a day really helps!

Cigarette smoking
Smoking constricts blood vessels and causes a more intense, prolonged flash. STOP!

Stress
Learn relaxation techniques such deep abdominal breathing or take a yoga class. Have massages on a regular basis.

Having kept a journal and identified your own triggers, why don't you now take a pro-active stance and do these two key activities:

31

1. Prepare Your Response

We often feel that everyone can see our hot flash. Look in the mirror during a flash. Is it as noticeable as you thought? Is your face red or glowing, perspiring or sweaty? Rehearse what your response will be when someone asks and you have to say, "Yes, I am having a hot flash." It will be a catharsis for your soul to be open and honest; really!

2. Join A Support Group

Talking about your experience in a safe environment is empowering. You can motivate yourself and others by the discovery of positive aspects of menopause.

FITNESS OPTIONS

Numerous studies have documented that exercise improves the circulation and allows your body to tolerate temperature changes, as well as cool down faster. Exercise lessens the frequency and intensity of hot flashes by reducing stress and improving regulation of body temperature through sweating. Exercise stimulates the endocrine system including the ovaries and adrenal glands; thus increasing the amount of estrogen circulating in the blood and decreasing frequency of hot flashes.

Exercise also activates the release of certain hormones within the brain called endorphins–which produce a sense of well-being during and after exercise. This improves the quality of sleep, too.

Cardiorespiratory exercise and stress reduction exercises such as yoga, stretching and relaxation seem to be ideal choices to diminish frequency and intensity of hot flashes.

Cardiorespiratory exercise is any activity that is rhythmic, continuous and uses large muscles of the body. It is any activity that lasts for a period of twenty to thirty minutes. The selection of the activity is the key to your success. It should be an activity that interests you and that you enjoy. Have you always wanted to be a dancer? Who says you can't take up the art of dancing–including belly, country, jazz or ballroom?

Make sure whatever exercise you choose is convenient to do. Do not add another stress in your life with a fitness activity. Convenience means it fits your lifestyle. Do not sign up for a class that begins at 5:00p.m., in a studio across town, that requires you have to drive through rush hour traffic to get there. If you are not a morning person, do not commit to a 6:00a.m. class. Many of my clients live by their appointment book. If they schedule an appointment with me, it becomes convenient to keep the appointment.

Cardiorespiratory activities include:

> **Dancing**
> **Walking**
> **Cycling**
> **Rollerskating**
> **Rollerblading**
> **Swimming**
> **Cross country skiing**
> **Stair Climbing**

Stretching exercises, as well as yoga, when done on a regular basis, will ease chronically tensed muscles and allow your body to relax. Slow abdominal breathing done at least once a day is helpful in reducing the stress that may trigger your hot flashes. You can manage your hot flashes!

How to have an intense hot flash . . .

*It is a <u>hot</u>, <u>humid</u> day in July and you're <u>rushing</u>
home. You and your significant other finally are off
to have dinner at the new, hot spot that features <u>Tex-
Mex cuisine</u>. You are wearing the dress you "just
had to have," even though you didn't try it on or see
the fabric tag—<u>100% polyester</u>. For openers, you
have a <u>double margarita</u>. In the middle of your
devourment of the <u>"large, hot</u> & <u>spicy</u> special" you
get into a heated <u>argument</u> with your partner.
Finally, to celebrate the resolving of the <u>conflict</u>, you
seal the evening with an <u>Irish coffee</u>, double <u>sugar</u>
and a <u>cigarette</u>. On the way home you think to
yourself, wow, I've sure had a lot of hot flashes
tonight! Wonder why?*

*P.S. "Dear Mother Adelaide, I sincerely apologize
for my expression of disgust all those years when
every time beads of sweat appeared on your brow,
you feverishly fanned with any object within arm's
reached and shouted, I'm having a hot flash!"*

*"In the long run we shape our
lives and we shape ourselves.
The process never ends . . .
and the choices we make are
ultimately our own
responsibility."*

ELEANOR ROOSEVELT

CHAPTER TWO

Body Weight and Diet

(The D Word)

Y ou have the family curse . . . a pot belly." (Mother)
"Your hips are so narrow. You're built just like a boy."
(Boyfriend's Mother)

"Don't worry, you will eventually have breasts. It takes time." (Grandmother Marie)

"Please God, don't let this tissue paper fall out of my bathing suit!!!" (Me at the pool)

"Honest, Grandma. My shoe size is 7. New shoes are always tight!" (Me at age 15)

"As you get older, you'll need more meat on those bones." (Mother's friend)

"You're not fat. Besides, voluptuous women are sexy—something to hold on to." (Boyfriend)

"I passed the pencil test. My breasts are so high they can't hold a pencil underneath." (Me at age 35)

"It's never too early to start wearing a girdle. It keeps everything nice and tight." (Girlfriend at age 16)

"My face isn't fat—those are dimples in my cheek." (Me looking at my 30 year-old photograph)

"Oh, I remember when I had a shape like yours." (Aunt Irene)

"When I was married, I wore a perfect size 6." (Mother)

"You can never be too rich or too thin." (Unknown, attributable to many!)

The Body. That which distinguishes me from you. It is constantly changing. Changing, whether or not we initiate the change, or sit back and watch the change happen. Body stereotypes and influences come from individuals and outside sources like magazines, films and television. Some we believe and some we just don't accept, but some do affect us.

Let me share with you how I came to deal with body weight gains, shifts, and the D word–DIET. Take this chance to reflect back in your own mind, about where your ideas and images about weight and diet originate. I just bet that you will discover some of the same situations that I faced. Do you think that just because I am writing this book, I was always athletic and physically fit? Wrong! I received an award in high school for compiling the longest list of excuses for skipping PE class. In fact, I could have had a successful business–writing creative pleas for all my classmates. I just was not into sweat. My joy while growing up was retiring to my room with a good book. Yes, I was the nerd-type who looked at sports and physical activity as waste of my time, and certainly beneath my intellectual endeavors. I was a skinny kid with the "cursed Myers pot belly" that frequently was cause for speculation that I was pregnant. My feet were invariably too big, my body straight up and down except for that pot belly and I had no hips but tiny, firm breasts that stood "at attention." However, I did enjoy ice skating in the winter wonderland of my hometown. Some of my fondest memories were of the rink that my father would make in our back yard. Mastering figure eight's and skating backward were skills I had that filled me with pride.

My mother Adelaide had been a professional dancer before her marriage. Everyone in St. Paul remembers the day when Bo Jangles, that famous Hollywood hoofer known for his tap dance with Shirley Temple, came to town and invited eight-year old "little Adelaide" onto the stage to dance with him. Bo called her "Little Mis' Bo Jangles" and Mother was so proud of that nickname she acquired. People always referred to that whenever the "good old days" were discussed.

The highlight of her dance career was performing in a trio with Dorothy Dandridge and being invited to move to Hollywood. Grandmother Marie would not hear of such a thing. I don't think Mother ever stopped wondering "what would have happened if I had gone?" So instead, she put her creative energy into raising six children and settled for producing and choreographing hometown theater productions.

Mother had always wanted to play the piano, so her desire was passed down to me as an ultimatum. From age ten to sixteen, I took piano lessons and hated every moment. Around the age of fifteen, I really began being interested in dancing myself. But when I expressed my desire to Mother, she said, "You can't dance when you are forty–but you can play the piano." So my piano lessons continued.

I began nursing school in a flurry of study and work after graduating from college. My body was not an issue. It remained the same until I had my son Michael at age twenty-three. My breasts became fuller and now, I had hips–this was okay by me! These were changes I watched happen without any intervention–like diet or exercise. Nursing is an occupation that is stressful, and exercise was the last thing I wanted to do when I came home from the hospital. So, my biggest exercise was lifting food to my mouth, pushing away from the dinner table, walking to living room and turning on the TV. Oh, yes I forgot. This was before remote control, so I did get more exercise as I got up to switch the TV channel. This was my routine from age twenty-three to twenty-seven. I was transported by a low energy, 5'4" body that weighed 148 pounds.

In January 1969, I made my first visit to San Francisco. Liking almost everything about the City by the Bay, in November 1969, I moved here permanently. By that time, I was a single parent, with no job, no apartment, but a vision that San Francisco was where I should be. I had saved enough money to go on a sabbatical–a leave from traditional nursing–to explore new options. San Francisco was the heart of the beginning of the human potential movement, and I jumped right in. (Jumping in literally being some of the first exercise in my life!) I took Tai Chi, studied Esalen massage, experienced my first dance class as a twenty-seven year old in a ballet studio with kids who watched me struggle through each plié. A year later, since I needed to get back to the real world of securing funds to pay rent and eat, etc . . . it was time to go back to work. But, I just couldn't go back to traditional nursing.

By January 1970, I discovered that I was in a body that felt and moved totally differently. I felt and looked better than I ever had before; and it all came from moving this body. MOVING! So how about a center with body-based approaches to well-being–that's what I want to open. That will be my nursing career and the vision of why I came to San Francisco in the first place–self-discovery and new beginning. In 1971, my Creative Bodywork Center opened. We moved to a larger location in 1975 that offered classes in yoga, Tai Chi, exercise (before it was called aerobics), and massage. So I went from a sedentary youth and young adult nurse to a vibrant, physically fit and firm visionary ready to propagate the benefits of body-based approaches to well-being. It all began when I started to MOVE this body!

Have you ever asked yourself–Why does my body have to change–gaining and losing weight, shifting around? Do you remember if you ever have loved the body you once had? Do you worry that it will not remain the same? Does your mind's eye see the body of yesterday, but your outer eyes see the body of today and the future?

Yes, you are normal. Your body has changed as you progress through mid-life and menopause. It is a combination of decreased activity, decreased lean muscle mass, the slowing down of our endocrine glands (thyroid and pituitary) and that we metabolize food at a slower rate. So what can we do about these mid-life and menopausal weight gains and shifts? EXERCISE. It stimulates the endocrine glands, it stimulates your metabolism, increases your lean muscle mass and reduces your body fat. The fitness choice of exercise is important for best results in managing your weight. Here are some suggestions based upon my years of experience.

Strength Training

Leanness. It is our eternal wish at all times. Is it elusive? No! In order to acquire this body composition, strength training is the key to tricking the biological clock. Lean muscle was what described our body composition in our twenties and thirties. How do we acquire lean muscle again? By asking our muscles to do more than they are accustomed to. A progressive load on the muscles creates the muscle density to increase your caloric requirements. Weight training is the key for lean body mass and should be a component of your exercise program. Some specific descriptions of an ideal program are found in Part Three.

Balance in our life is essential as we age. The way to have balance is to have a plan based on our goals of what we wish to achieve. If we want to increase our metabolism, we must plan a program that addresses those needs. Strength training combined with nutrition–what we put into our bodies–that all contributes to our body composition. The combination of nutrition and exercise is important to reduce body fat, increase lean muscle and feed ourselves with wholesome food. We usually look at what we take in as the key. During menopause, we must look at how we metabolize, in other words, how efficient are our bodies in processing what we take in. What energy expenditure will it take to increase our metabolic factory–our muscles?

Endurance activities that involve raising the heart rate for a length of time are important for the reduction of body fat and weight control. This exercise format is usually referred to as aerobic exercises. Changing our body composition is the key to losing weight. We want to decrease our body fat–with cardiorespiratory exercise and increase our lean muscle with strength exercises. Fat reductions by cardiorespiratory exercises include ones that use large muscles, are rhythmic and continue over a time. Please refer to Part Three for some specific exercises in these categories.

Where's The Fat?

Determining where the fat is accumulating on your body is important in determining certain disease risks. Fat that accumulates around your waist and lower abdomen is metabolically more active, and is frequently associated with increased risk of coronary heart disease, hypertension, diabetes, high blood cholesterol and possibly breast cancer. There is another incentive for your fitness–by exercising and losing weight, you can significantly reduce your risk of developing many of these diseases.

Learning to eat for health and well-being should be our emphasis at this time. Now we can look at a new plan for optimal nutrition based on improving the quality of life–how we feel emotionally; what foods trigger mood swings; hot flashes; what food affects bone density; what food influences our cardiorespiratory risk; what food alters our cancer risk. We now have a new impetus to our diet, and to eating; it is one that not only satisfies our taste buds, but also serves our life. It is now more than counting calories. It is putting the ideal calories into our bodies to affect our longevity and health status today and tomorrow. Eating for life is our plan now.

Fat In Means Fat On

A diet minus the fat? Let's begin to think of a diet sparsely sprinkled with fat. Reducing fat is an important key to keeping weight under control. Fat consists of twice the amount of calories per gram more than carbohydrates and protein. Reducing fat in your diet is a major health issue. High fat diets have been linked to heart disease, high blood pressure, cancer of the breast, ovaries, uterus and colon. The American Heart Association (AHA) recommends to get <u>no more than thirty percent of your calories from fat</u>. Cutting down on red meat sharply reduces fat intake. Choosing fish and chicken is ideal. Look at every meat portion on your plate as a side dish rather than the main entree.

Protein

How much protein do we need at this time in our life? Too much protein causes urinary excretion of calcium–depleting that essential calcium from the bones leading to bone loss. That fact is an important consideration as we are looking at risk for osteoporosis at menopause. High dietary protein in excess converts to fat. This is another reason to examining your diet at this time of life, based on how it affects your entire well-being. Excess weight and reduction of bone density should be our concern when considering the amount of protein in our diet. It is recommended that we get <u>no more than fifteen percent of our calories from protein.</u>

Carbohydrates

Think green and wholesome. These are the life of our diet, the carbohydrates. Of course all will not be green, but you have heard it before. Eat at least five servings of fruits and vegetables; and for nutritional value and eating variety, visualize a mixture of colors. Green broccoli, red apple, yellow squash, orange fruit, white cauliflower. Thinking in a variety of colors is one helpful way to plan your daily intake and will balance the nutrients of value. Add to the list complex carbohydrates such as breads, pasta, grains, beans and rice. This is your most intake of your diet. "Carbs" are our main source of energy. <u>At least sixty percent of your diet should be carbohydrates</u>. This is your main course. Fat and protein are the side dishes to main course carbohydrates.

The Heart of the Matter

As estrogen decreases in our bodies, we are at a higher risk of heart disease. To live a full, healthy life, our diet is extremely important. High levels of fat in animals and some dairy products suggests that the change to a vegetarian lifestyle is one great way to achieve lower that fat intake. Reducing the fat in our diet according to the AHA is the best way to decrease our risk to heart disease. This, along with a regular exercise program is recommended to considerably decrease the risk of this disease that we were protected from with our higher levels of estrogen.

"Fad" Diets

A quick fix "fad diet" is tempting during menopausal time when the jeans are too tight and the exercises we did when were young do not give quick results. The diet that will make you lose ten pounds in two weeks . . . yeah, right! This is a time to get professional advice about your diet. It is time to invest time in studying sound nutrition advice from a registered dietitian. They can assist you in planning eating that will eliminate those "not needed calories" and allow you maintain or reduce your body weight based on reliable principles. Remember, nutrition AND exercise combined are most beneficial for eliminating body weight gains/shifts.

The attitude component of fluctuating body weight changes can cause feelings such as "I don't even like my body. I can't do anything about these weight gains." These are the kinds of feelings that causes stress. Stress that can trigger an urge to eat. Eating that causes us to gain weight. A vicious cycle. Know that you can make changes with your body with exercise, nutrition and attitude. Take the steps you are learning in this book. Find your favorite stress buster and do it on a regular basis. Be the master of your changes rather than the victim. Studies show that active women weigh thirty percent less than sedentary women, even though both groups eat about the same amount of food.

What to Remember About Managing Body Weight Gains / Shifts

FITNESS OPTIONS

* Cardiorespiratory exercise 3-5 times a week.
* Strength Training 2-3 times per week.
* Dance (any variety).

LIFESTYLE OPTIONS

* Get sound nutritional advice.
* Read the latest books.
* Eat carbohydrates with protein and fat on the side.
* Make a goal of 60% carbohydrates, 25 % fats, 15% protein.
* Avoid fad diets.
* Practice stress reduction.

Know that your body knows what is right for it.

"Take a stand."

"The backbone of the family."

"Spineless!"

"I can't stand this any longer."

"Get off my back!"

"Carry the weight on your shoulders."

"The straw that broke the camel's back."

"Stand up under the pressure."

"My life is caving in."

"I will back you up."

THE DIALOGUE OF POSTURE

CHAPTER 3

Posture &
Osteoporosis

Dateline: March 1993
Post-Ken Dychtwald's Age Wave Institute
New York City

Leora does the Big Apple! I was fortunate and able to attend noted author and speaker Ken Dychtwald's dynamic presentation of research findings and insights into the aging of America. I stayed on for a few days to "escape" and enjoy the electric and eclectic city. As I was walking down Broadway, I came upon a dance studio. As I climbed the stairs up to the third floor, I was propelled back into my own dance studio days of the 1970s–an arena of dancers stretching and warming up for class decked out in worn tights, leggings, broken-in shoes and self-assured attitudes. Looking through the studio's schedule, I found a class that I figured I could handle–a little dance and exercise combination–should be stimulating, but not too complicated.

At the beginning of the session, it was announced that the regular teacher (whom I was told was superb) was ill and there would be a substitute. The sub walks in the room and she is at least fifty-five years old with a slight limp. Great, I'm thinking, my one dance class in New York and I get her.

What can she teach? I have noticed that as we mature, a phenomenon frequently occurs–where what we assume is going to be a disappointing experience turns out to be quite incredible and enriches our life. It's as if our life becomes an enjoyable classroom. I was about to have such an experience. The instructor starts her music, which turns out to be Annie Lennox (my favorite) and I begin to think that maybe this won't be so bad! Little did I know that this woman was to be one of my "teachers of life."

That woman gave me an unforgettable insight into posture. As a seasoned student and teacher of dance, she began by having us walk while she explained the meaning of our exercises. She had studied with the world renowned pantomime artist Marcel Marceau and relayed how he had portrayed life's posture. I will never forget what she shared. Namely, that in our youth, we walk with our head held high, excitedly looking for the opportunities that life has to offer. But as we age, we begin to look down with an attitude that life does not have much more to offer. The chest of youth that was thrust to the sky now begins to cave in, our shoulders round and our body no longer has a hopeful attitude. She shouted at us students, "Walk with the chest high to the heavens, with a sense of new horizons, new opportunities, new beginnings!" The "old" teacher that had walked in the room appeared younger with each movement, as her posture transformed her stride and she shared her "aged" words of wisdom.

Today, as I teach my fitness classes, I repeatedly challenge my students' posture with that image–the chest is the place of opportunity, the place to be lifted to the sky, a physical demonstration of an attitude of hope and expectation in our life. Posture is a recognizable characteristic denoting age. Just stand on a busy street corner and analyze a person's age by their posture. What you first recognize is most likely "attitude" age, not "chronological" age.

POSTURE

The spine is a structure of great precision, efficiency and architecture whose primary purpose is to maintain erect posture and allow movement of the head, neck and torso.

Before birth, our spine is C-curved. (Isn't it interesting to notice that as we age we begin to resume that posture.) After birth, around the third month of life, we want to see what is going on in the world, so we lift our head. This is a very important step for both us and our thrilled parents. Lifting our heads is our first look into the horizon with our eyes. At that time, our cervical curve (neck) is developed and we are able to balance our head. We are also able to contract the muscles behind our neck. By the age of nine months, we can crawl on our hands and knees, and the lumbar muscles (low back) and buttock muscles can contract. By ten months' age, after crawling up on furniture, we are ready to discover the world. We begin to walk, then run into this world and the lumbar curve is developed. As our parents discovered, there are no boundaries to our explorations and there is great excitement with each discovery we make. So we go from the C-curve in utero, to looking up into the horizon, creating our neck curve and having a need to move out into the world, we begin to walk and create the lumbar curve. As we are anatomically created, so is our purpose in life. Looking to the horizon and moving forward . . . the true function of the spine we must remember as we age.

When I began my quest to challenge aging and menopause, I looked far and wide for information on posture and came up dry. I found plenty of references to the old axiom "just stand up straight." Posture is so much more than just standing up straight. Excellent posture creates a new dialogue with your body; especially when followed up with effective action. So what is the strategy for a posture that gives us total support, structure and carries us into the second half our lives?

The choices for optimal, functional posture at any age include: attitude, balance, strength, and flexibility.

Attitude

Yes, I believe posture is a big part attitude–a person's age is determined by the attitude of their posture–the position or bearing of the body and how we interact with the world. With each thought there is a reciprocal body response. This is the importance of our thoughts which are responsible for our attitudes. Attitudes are recognized as feelings. Feelings change with the posture as well as change the posture. Try this exercise.

Find an area where you can stroll. Get a brisk walk going and swing your arms freely and easy and breathe. Lift the chest to the sky as your shoulders naturally roll back and down. Feel the shoulder blades pinching together giving support to the uplifted chest. Lift the chin slightly as the eyes look forward. Inhale and exhale freely. **Notice how you feel.** Now slow the arm movements and begin to lower the eyes and chin looking downward. Roll the shoulders forward and downward and allow the breathing to become shallow. **Notice how you feel.** Was there an age shift with the two postures? When did you feel young? When did you feel old? How did your breathing affect how you felt? What emotions came up in each posture? In what position did you feel strong? Weak? In what position did you feel hopeful? Despondent? This exercise demonstrates your personal response to posture.

An habitual attitude creates an habitual body posture. This exercise is for you to explore the body attitude you wish to carry into the second half of your life. How do you what to feel in the second half of your life? How do you what to carry your body? How do you what to be supported? How do you want to stand? Note your response to each position and observe your feelings throughout the day. Notice if your posturing is affecting your feelings.

Balance

Every muscle has an opposite muscle that counterbalances it. Opposing imbalance contributes to misalignment. Misalignment contributes to inefficiency. Imbalanced posture contributes to shallow breathing, stiff movement, shallow breathing and negative attitude. Our bodies now have areas that are strong and contracted and areas that are weak and stretched. Looking at the part of the body that constitutes inefficient or as referred to as "bad" posture, we see a contracted chest and front shoulders and opposing area that is stretched, the back and rear shoulders. We see the clear picture of muscles that need to be stretched and lengthened–the chest and front shoulders, as well as muscles that need to be strengthened and shortened–the back and rear shoulders.

These muscles, however, have become very comfortable in their misaligned states–they have worked long and hard to stay just like they are. To these muscles, this is the easiest position in which to remain. So you think to yourself–I must sit up straight. A few seconds later, the muscles reply–I'm not comfortable like this, I want my old posture back. Even though now you are misaligned, the body has found the path of least resistance and is very comfortable in a position that it knows best–a position it has designated as "balance". The body's posture represents repeated muscular contraction habits. Therefore it can be corrected with designed muscular contractions and flexibility designed for balance and efficiency.

In many instances, our fitness program has contributed to muscular imbalance such as:
–repeated chest presses without balance of middle back exercise; and, of course, daily life activities such as working at a desk or computer.

Strength

This is the conversation that strength exercises have with our body–this is where you should be, shoulders. This is where you should be, shoulder blades. This is the posture that was intended for you to be most proficient, balanced, have an expanded diaphragm and chest to breathe freely and efficiently. Strength exercises tell the muscles to contract. For posture, we need to strengthen or shorten the back muscles which are stretched or lengthened. When the chest is open and lifted, the opposing muscles need to contract to support that action. Those muscles are located in the back, specifically between the shoulder blades (rhomboids) and the lower back (erector spinae). Read the Fitness Options at the end of this chapter as well as Part 3—Leora's Complete Exercise Guide for additional tips.

Flexibility

Flexibility exercises tell the muscles that have been long contracted to stretch and lengthen. When the balance of strong contracted muscles in the back occurs, the opposing muscle groups have to reciprocate by lengthening to create body balance. When we talk about posture, the muscles in the chest and front shoulders need to lengthen. Growing up in the snowy land of Minnesota, I enjoyed this exercise as a child, never thinking it would be one of the most effective exercises for expansion of the chest and shoulders (and prevention of osteoporosis in my mid-life)!

<u>SNOW ANGELS</u>
Lie on a bench or place pillows under your spine so that your chest can be elevated off the floor. Knees are bent.
1) Extend arms to ceiling directly over the chest with palms facing in.
2) Slowly extend arms over head. Stop when arms are at ears.
3) Slowly open palms to ceiling and sweep arms to side.
4) Pause when arms are extended to side and you feel the stretch across your chest.

5) Draw arms to side and up to starting position.

6) Repeat 8-10 times. Lengthen pause up to 15-20 seconds.

OSTEOPOROSIS

Posture is a tremendous concern as we age. Maybe, those who always told us to "Stand up straight" were experiencing the posture they related to old age and wanted to assure we did not have to suffer the same recourse. When we approach menopause, we are also concerned with osteoporosis. Where posture is a function of muscle condition and spinal health, osteoporosis deals with bones and bone density. However, amazingly, the mention of osteoporosis in our society gives an instant mental picture of a bent over woman–the posture of menopause! **Thus, these two distinct physical issues–posture and osteoporosis–become implicitly linked.**

Osteoporosis. What picture comes to your mind when you see that word? How about a short, elderly, frail woman, hunched forward, with her rounded back walking cautiously along with a cane? That is a scenario we all cringe at; and hope that it will not happen to us. Simply, osteoporosis means porous bone and a change in the bone structure itself.

Calcium

Bone is a living tissue constantly being torn down (resorption) and replaced with new bone (remodeling). Resorption and remodeling are ongoing balanced functions of our bones. These processes also help keep a constant level of calcium in the bloodstream. Calcium is critical to make the bone dense, as well as essential for the forceful beating of your heart and the clotting of your blood. Ninety percent of the body's calcium is stored in the bones and teeth and helps maintain your bones' strength. Your bones also serve as a calcium storage space for other tissues in the body. Our bones keep increasing in density until we are about thirty-five years old.

Estrogen appears to improve the absorption of calcium. However, in menopause, the hormone estrogen becomes decreased in our system. The loss of estrogen influences the metabolism of calcium, causing an increase in resorption compared to the remodeling.

The amount of calcium in your diet is extremely important. It is never too early to begin focusing on your calcium intake. Your peak bone mass (achieved at age thirty-five,) will affect your bone density as you age. Thus, the more bone mass you have at age thirty-five will directly affect the likelihood of developing osteoporosis.

The normal recommended intake of 1,000 mg of calcium per day will not prevent osteoporosis in the postmenopausal woman. This illustrates the importance of a balanced diet rich in calcium throughout our life especially before age thirty-five. The National Institute of Health's Consensus Panel on Osteoporosis recommends:

-1,000 mg of calcium daily for
    premenopausal women.
-1,000 mg of calcium daily for post menopausal
    women taking estrogen
-1,500 mg of calcium daily for postmenopausal
    women not taking estrogen.

Calcium derived from food is the best source as they are in an absorbable form. However, concern for caloric intake usually indicates taking calcium supplements. Calcium carbonate is the least expensive, but it is also the least well absorbed. Calcium citrate is more expensive, but results in better absorption. It is best when taken in small amounts during the day. Certain foods interfere with the absorption of calcium and should be avoided within two hours of taking supplemental calcium–excessive fiber, aluminum (found in antacids) and caffeine (in chocolate, tea, coffee and sodas). Vitamin D 400 IU should be taken with the calcium supplements as it aids the absorption from the intestinal tract. Numerous

Alternate Calcium Sources

Calcium can also be obtained from sources other than milk products. The following foods contain at least 250 mg. of calcium per serving indicated below:

5 medium sardines, with bones (2 1/2 oz.)
1/2 cup canned salmon, with bones
5 oz. mackerel, canned
9 oz. tofu (must be processed with a calcium salt)
4 oz. almonds
1/4 cup tahini
2 cups baked beans or pork and beans
7 corn tortillas (treated with lime or calcium carbonate, as is masahanna)
5 medium oranges
1 1/2 cups broccoli, fresh, cooked
1 1/2 cups turnip greens, cooked
2 cups bok choy, collard or dandelion greens, cooked
3 cups kale or mustard greens, cooked
2 Tbsp. blackstrap molasses

supplements contain this Vitamin D and it can also be acquired by exposure to the sun.

Other minerals important in bone building are:
Phosphorus is the second most prevalent mineral in bones. However an excess of phosphorous, relative in relation to calcium, can lead to bone loss. Since our typical U.S. diet is high in phosphorus, a supplementation is not necessary. At the same time, avoid "soda drinks" (artificially carbonated)

which are high in phosphorous and low in calcium, as is red meat . . . a good reason to give up the hamburger and soda! Magnesium is the third most prevalent mineral in the bones. Sugar and alcohol consumption increase urinary excretion of magnesium, leading to magnesium deficiency, which impairs utilization of calcium for bone building. Interesting note: chocolate is high in magnesium . . . maybe those chocolate cravings are a sign of magnesium deficiency! Suggested daily dose is at least 300mg/day.

Prevention

The ultimate question always is–can diet and exercise alone prevent osteoporosis?

If you have examined the risk factor chart (see page 63) and find that you are at high risk for osteoporosis, evidence suggests that the combination of exercise, plus a diet high in calcium and estrogen together, gives the best results in stopping bone loss. Exercise and calcium alone may slow the rate of bone loss, but the addition of estrogen is the only medication that has been clinically shown to prevent osteoporosis. To be effective in stopping bone loss, hormone replacement therapy (HRT) must be started within six years of menopause. The greatest degree of bone loss occurs during the first few years after menopause, and studies indicate that you need to remain on HRT until bone loss begins to slow down naturally, approximately around age sixty-five. As you can see, this is a long-term commitment.

Hormones will only prevent accelerated loss of bone that occurs after menopause. They will not restore the bone to premenopausal density levels. For women unable to take the hormone estrogen (such as those with estrogen-dependent breast cancer or fearing cancer and side effects of estrogen), there are pharmaceutical alternatives for preventing osteoporosis. They include calcitonin, given by injection, which has been shown to inhibit bone resorption and be highly effective in replacing bone mass; as well as anabolic steroids (hormones related to testosterone) that prevent bone loss and increase total body calcium. Natural progesterone, found in wild Mexican yams and soybeans can also help to build bone tissue and aid in the prevention of osteoporosis.

The most important choices we can make surround our fitness and lifestyle options. The keys to optimal posture and the prevention of osteoporosis throughout life are balance, strength, flexibility. Here are my suggestions.

FITNESS OPTIONS

Strength Training

Studies indicate that high intensity strength training improves bone density. When muscles contract, they pull on the bone where the muscle attaches, stimulating the bone to conserve calcium and making the bone stronger, more dense. For years, it was thought that only weight bearing exercises like walking or running could have an effect on building strong bones.

Now, looking at the importance of the areas in which we wish to have a bone density increase, one can understand the importance of a total body workout of one set per body part, eight to twelve repetitions of high loads. High loads mean using enough weight that does not allow you to do more than twelve repetitions. Only by using high loads will you have the intense pull on the bone that will make a difference in your bone density.

The following exercise strengthens the back using body weight and resistance machines. This exercise should be included in your regular exercise regimen.

Chest Expansion
This exercise stretches the muscles in the chest and shoulders.
Stand with arms at side and feet are hip distance apart and knees are slightly bent.

1) Stretch arms back and clasp hands
2) Exhale and straighten arms and begin to raise arms upward. Keep body upright; do not bend forward.
3) Hold this position for 5 seconds.
4) Unclasp your hands and rest arms at side
5) Repeat exercise 3 times.
-Don't raise shoulders
-Breathe deeply

Machines or Free Weights?

One study conducted on bone density suggested that free weights training had more benefits than machines. Weight machines are designed to isolate the muscle being exercised while stabilizing the rest of the body. Example: when doing a seated shoulder press on a machine, your body is positioned in a way that your back and legs are stable and all work is in the shoulders. In a standing shoulder press, the abdominals, lower back and legs are the stabilizers–which means they have to work just to keep you standing upright. You are also working on balance, an important aspect of life. Furthermore, a standing press is more "life functional"–resembling activities we do every day.

The American College of Sports Medicine recommends the following program for developing muscular strength:
Frequency: 2-3 times per week with a 48 hour rest period between workouts.
Duration:
8-12 repetitions. Sets: 1. Exercises: 8-10 (One exercise for each major muscle group.) Order: Work large to small muscles.

The following are exercises to strengthen the back using body weight and resistance machines.

<u>BACK EXTENSIONS</u>
Body weight exercises for back extension strengthen the back and promotes chest expansion. Move slowly through exercise. Do not hold breath. Breathe freely.

Level I

1) Kneel on floor on your hands and knees. Knees are apart and palms face forward under shoulders.
2) Shift the balance of weight to your right knee, as you lift your left leg straight behind you, parallel to the floor.
3) Feel balanced as you extend your right arm in front of you. Hold for 5-20 seconds.
4) Return to your original position and repeat with right leg and left arm.
5) Rest for 30 seconds.
6) Repeat 3-5 times.
Tips: Eyes are focused forward (not upward). Pelvis is parallel to floor. Do not lift hips. Extended arm and leg are strong and controlled.

Level II

Lie face down with arms at your side and head turned to one side. Legs and feet are relaxed.
1) Place arms at side with thumbs facing down.
2) Straighten legs and turn head face downward.
3) Inhale, then exhale and lift head face forward
4) Lift shoulders and trunk; lifting arms slightly off floor with fingertips toward your feet.
5) Hold this position 5-20 seconds, breathing deeply.
6) Return to original position and rest for 30 seconds.
Tips for success: Eyes look forward (not upward); do not raise your shoulders; and keep your legs active and strong during the exercise.

RESISTANCE EXERCISES

Using machines, if available, in a supervised gym or fitness center setting.
Cable Rows: Seated with back extended, knees bent and eyes forward. Weight: Sufficient to perform 12 repetitions. Exercise: Pull cable to waist, pause and slowly release to starting position.
Lat Pulls: Seated with back extended, feet on floor and cable directly over neck. Hands are placed on bar in a wide position with arms forming a "V." Weight: sufficient weight to

perform 12 repetitions. The last few reps should be a challenge. Exercise: pull bar to back of neck, pause and slowly release to starting position.

ABDOMINAL EXERCISES
Reverse Sit-ups--in typical abdominal sit-ups, the contraction begins by flexing the torso and rounding up from shoulders. This is the posture we are trying to avoid. Repeating sit-ups in this manner contribute to the rounded shoulder and contracted chest alignment. The emphasis in the reverse sit-up is to contract from the lower abdominal region.

Level I
Lying on back with knees bent and feet on floor, contract the abdominal muscles and slowly curl tail bone off the floor, hold contraction and slowly release. Repeat 8-10 times
Tips: do not press into floor with feet or arms to perform exercise. Lift your tail bone only. It is a small movement.

Level II
With arms at side, lift legs to ceiling in a hold perpendicular to floor, with a slight bend in the knees. Contract the lower abdominal region and curl tail bone off floor moving legs up vertically, pause and lower. Repeat exercise 8-10 times.
Tips: focus on legs staying perpendicular to floor and moving upward with each repetition. Do not press into floor with arms. Keep movements small and controlled.
Remember, this is a challenging exercise!

WEIGHT BEARING EXERCISES
Activities that consist of just you carrying your body weight around are defined as weight bearing exercises that place stress on the skeletal system stimulated by the muscular contractions. Sedentary women who avoid weight-bearing exercise increase the risk of developing osteoporosis. Activities include dancing, aerobics, stair climbing, racket sports, and walking three to five times a week for 20-30 minutes.

Swimming

It is only recently that studies indicate swimming may increase bone density. The factor important to understand how swimming improves muscle strength and flexibility (and bone) is the resistant effect of the water when swimming. The use of aquatic props such as paddles, webbed gloves, flotation barbells, vests and belts increases the resistance factor even more. Most research has been conducted on lap swimmers, although there is value to aquatic exercise especially for individuals that are overweight, have joint problems or are arthritic. Swimming adds an enjoyable variety to your workout plan with the added benefit of increasing bone density.

LIFESTYLE OPTIONS

Body Weight

This is not a time to be too thin. Women with less than fifteen percent body fat put less stress on the bones that results in bones not becoming as dense. Also, they have less fat cells that continue after menopause to convert hormones into estrogen. Estrogen protects against bone loss. Thin women have less estrogen than heavier women. Being overweight increases the risk of fractures as it puts too much stress on the bones. See Chapter Two for "diet options."

Alcohol and Caffeine

Both increase bone loss. They interfere with calcium and vitamin D metabolism in the liver and act as diuretics, increasing the amount of calcium excreted in the urine. The more alcohol and caffeine that you consume on a regular basis, the higher incidence of developing osteoporosis. The good news is that recent studies indicate that one to two cups of coffee or tea, a glass of wine or beer, or 1 1/2 ounces of hard liquor consumed within a 24-hour period is probably not harmful to bone density.

Smoking

Women who smoke go through menopause earlier than non-smokers. Because they are without the protective effect of estrogen for a longer time, this is a risk factor for osteoporosis. Smoking also directly affects bone loss even at the normal menopause age.

Risk Factors for Osteoporosis

GENETIC OR MEDICAL

* Caucasian or Asian race.
* Female relatives with osteoporosis.
* Early menopause (natural before 40 or
        surgical).
* Daily use of cortisone; over 2 grains of
        thyroid medication.
* Being thin.
* Kidney disease with dialysis.

LIFESTYLE

* Smoking.
* High alcohol use.
* High caffeine use.
* High protein diet.
* Low calcium intake.
* Lack of exercise.

*"Life shrinks or expands in
proportion to one's courage."*

ANAIS NIN

CHAPTER 4

Breast Cancer

Dateline: February 2, 1994
"The Doctor's Office"
San Francisco, California

"Leora, there is a lump in your right breast. I need to refer you to see a breast surgeon."

Those simple words, when put together in a sentence and directed at you–are words that vibrate like a deep echo in your heart. Those words are words that someone else is supposed to hear . . . never you! It was two days before my 52nd birthday. I was going through my yearly Pap smear, mammogram and medical examination–a "body check-in" that I do annually as I approach another year in my life. I never attach any feelings or contemplations to the process. It's just the thing to do "on a regular basis." I'm sure it is a carry-over from my nursing days. I never expect to hear anything but light, casual conversation with the medical practitioner performing the exam and a perfunctory, "Everything looks fine, Leora. See you next year." Today, the script has taken a surprising turn. I swallow hard and say, "Are you sure?"

"Leora, feel this," is the response, and my fingers are guided to the suspect tissue. I really don't want to touch this invader, but I do, and yes, I do feel something. I am embarrassed to admit it feels different than usual. I am ashamed, that I, Leora

Myers, R.N. and health advocate, do not do regular breast exams. Why? Because like so many women, I've also feared feeling what I am now forced to feel–a lump in my breast.

My life has instantly changed. I feel as if I am walking in slow motion; disconnected; my body not feeling like mine; feeling invaded with "the lump"; wanting to touch my breast, but not wanting to touch "it," yet knowing I must deal with "it." So I make the call to my HMO (health maintenance organization) and hear, "The first appointment open is in two weeks, do you wish to take it?" I think, this must be a joke, lady, I have a lump in my breast! "Yes, I'll take it." I guess I'm in no big hurry to know, anyway.

Two days later, February 4, 1994, "Happy Birthday To Me." The day dawned beautiful and sunny for my luncheon celebration. My students shower me with laughter, encouragement and beautiful gifts; not knowing about the dark spot in my heart and the invader in my breast. I come to the last package to open and how revealing–it is a red lace bra, made for two breasts, of course. The irony of it all, as I joined the howls screaming, "How sexy! Thank you so much!" but inside thinking, you all have no idea how significant this gift is.

As I load the gifts into the car, I make a decision. I can't wait two weeks to get an appointment with a specialist. I need to see the best breast surgeon right now. I call my friend Dr. Joan Saxton, and I get the name that I need. Thank goodness, the specialist can see me right away. My mammogram is sent to his office.

February 7, 1994. The doctor walks in with my chart, sits down and says, "Leora, what exactly do you feel in your breast?" He goes on to explain how he will check my breasts and precisely what he is looking for. In my soul, I knew that whatever the outcome of this exam was, I had found the right person. He was sensitive and respectful to this moment in my life. If this tissue is malignant, I trust this physician with my care. The examination is complete.

"Well, Leora this is it, you will leave this office with your answer."
"I am ready," I reply.
"Leora, the tissue is normal."

Many women are given the opposite diagnosis from the one that I receive–"You have breast cancer."
Even though I did not have breast cancer, I have had three clients diagnosed within the last two years. My personal fitness training and classes have taken on another aspect of emotional support and listening, as these strong women faced the fear that comes with the diagnosis.

Breast cancer is the most common, and the most feared form of cancer among women. If you have close relatives, especially your mother or sister who have cancer of the breast, you are at the highest risk of developing it yourself. However, more recently, researchers are seeing that the majority of women developing this disease have no family history of the disease.

The following information should alert every woman to develop a **breast cancer monitoring plan**, as well as be aware of the risk factors that contribute to this deadly condition.

Age
Women over age fifty account for the majority of patients developing breast cancer. Approximately three fourths of the women are over fifty years old and the average age of diagnosis is sixty-two years old.

Race
White (Caucasian) people are at greater risk than dark-skinned individuals.

Delayed Childbearing
Women who had their children after age thirty; or have no

children, have greater risk than women who had their first child at age eighteen.

Family History
Fifteen to twenty percent of all breast cancer patients have a history of a close (immediate) family member diagnosed with breast cancer.

Obesity & Dietary Factors
Obesity increases the risk of developing breast cancer along with a high fat diet. Studies show a five to ten time difference in deaths due to breast cancer between countries with low fat diets and those with high fat diets. Dietary fat, along with caffeine, alcohol and low levels of Vitamin A and Vitamin E have been linked to higher incidences of breast cancer.

Dense Breast Tissue
Women with dense or firmer breast tissue are at higher risk than those with less dense or non-fatty breast tissue.

Breast Feeding
Breast feeding decreases the risks of breast cancer.

Radiation
Exposure to radiation increases risk of developing breast cancer. However, it is important to note that the amount of radiation you are exposed to during a mammogram is minimal and should not be a concern.

FITNESS Reduces the Risk of Breast Cancer!

Preliminary studies suggest a substantial decrease in the risk of breast cancer in women who exercise regularly. A study of exercise and breast cancer conducted by Harvard epidemiologist Rose Frisch also indicated that those who work at physically demanding jobs were less likely to have had breast cancer than those with sedentary jobs. Exercise, whether at work or in play, appears to reduce the risk of breast cancer.

Knowing our risk factors and addressing them through changes with our fitness and lifestyle patterns is the best method we can use to ease our anxiety–as well as take an active role in monitoring our breast health. Most importantly, early detection of breast cancer has the highest survival rate. Here are some activities for you; specifically surrounding breast cancer prevention.

FITNESS OPTIONS

*Exercise a minimum of three to six hours a week. Use a balanced program of strength training, aerobics and flexibility. Please refer to Part Three–Leora's Complete Exercise Guide for details.

LIFESTYLE OPTIONS

* Reduce fat in diet.
* Reduce caffeine.
* Moderate alcohol intake.
* Do a monthly breast self-exam beginning at age twenty. (See following chart.)
* Have your first mammogram at between the ages of thirty-five and thirty-nine to establish a baseline. Then, have a mammogram every two years between the ages of forty and forty-nine and one every year after the age of fifty.

How To Do Breast Self-Exam

1. Lie down and put a pillow under your right shoulder. Place your right arm behind your head. (See Figure 1.)

2. Use the finger pads of your three middle fingers on your hand to feel for lumps or thickening. Your finger pads are the top third of each finger. (See Figure 2.)

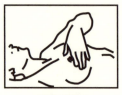

FIGURE 1

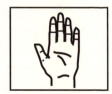

FIGURE 2

3. Press firmly enough to know how your breast feels If you are not sure how hard to press, ask your health care provider. Or try to copy the way your health care provider uses his or her finger pads during a breast exam. Learn what your breast feel like most of the time. A firm ridge in the lower curve of each breast is normal.

4. Move your finger pads over your breast in a methodical pattern. One example of such a pattern is the inset Figure 3. Another way would be to move around your breast in concentric circles. Choose which way is best for you, and do it the same way each time. Using this set pattern will help you to make sure that you've gone over the entire breast area and to remember how your breast feels. Don't forget to also check your armpits for any lumps or thickening.

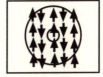

FIGURE 3

Other tips: For added safety, you might want to check your breast while standing in front of a mirror right after you do your breast self-exam each month. See if there are any changes in the way your breasts look: dimpling of the skin, changes in the nipple, or redness and swelling. Some women choose to do a breast self-exam while in the shower. Your soapy hands glide well over your wet skin, making it easy to check how your breasts feel.

Source: American Cancer Society; reprinted by permission.

"It's important to remember that falling estrogen levels are not the only cause of heart disease in older women. Diet, smoking, alcohol and stress all contribute importantly to this life-threatening illness. Heredity also plays a role. No amount of estrogen will protect you from heart disease if you have unhealthful lifestyle habits."

-KATHERINE O'HANLAN, M.D.,
Author, *Natural Menopause*

Heart Disease

Heart disease is the number one killer of American women. It strikes ten years later in females than in males; so that by age sixty, women face the same risk as men. Studies indicate that as the estrogen levels decrease during menopause, the chances of heart disease increase. The decline in estrogen is a precursor to coronary artery disease. Although no one knows the exact mechanism, at menopause there is an increase in total cholesterol. There is an increase in the harmful Low-Density Lipoproteins (LDL) cholesterol, while the protective High-Density Lipoproteins (HDL) cholesterol remains the same. Lack of estrogen directly affects the integrity of the blood vessels, predisposing them to cholesterol deposits and plaque formation. Research suggests that estrogen, in low doses, may improve blood flow to the heart, prevent constriction of the blood vessels and inhibit the rise in blood clotting factors. Remember, however, that hormone replacement therapy (HRT) is not without risk. Taking estrogen increases the risk of breast cancer. You should know the importance of HRT and its effects on life-threatening diseases like osteoporosis and heart disease. Your decision regarding HRT should come after weighing all the risks and benefits.

If your LDL cholesterol is elevated, your family history includes many who have heart disease and strokes, you are not exercising and have a poor diet–you may want to consider HRT. Please be aware of how many of these factors you can affect with lifestyle change. Your lifestyle choices not only reduce the risk of heart disease but also reduce risk of cancer.

The Risk Factors for Cardiovascular (Heart) Disease

* **Strong family history of cardiovascular disease** (parents, siblings) especially before age of sixty.
* Be aware of **your immediate family's health history**. Interview parents, grandparents regarding diet, exercise and physical conditions.
* Become conscious of **your own family's lifestyle choices.** Are you living the same way as your parents and grandparents?
* **Cigarette smoking** narrows the blood vessels, slows circulation throughout the body, and increases risk of heart attack.
* **Obesity** is the most important risk factor for heart disease due to the high amount of cholesterol and fat (lipid) in the bloodstream.
* **Elevated cholesterol** and triglycerides are carried in the blood by lipoproteins. High-density lipoproteins (HDL) remove excess cholesterol from bloodstream and send it to liver for excretion. They are called the "good cholesterol." Low-density lipoproteins (LDL) carry cholesterol from the liver to the various organs and deposit cholesterol in the blood vessels, the so-called "bad cholesterol."

* **Diabetes** increases blood sugar due to insufficient insulin, a hormone produced by the pancreas. Diabetes increases the risk of heart attacks.

* **Oral contraceptive** use past the age of thirty-five can cause the LDL level in the blood to rise due to the progestational agent in the Pill.

* **Hypertension** or high blood pressure is known as "the silent killer". It damages the blood vessel lining and promotes cholesterol build-up due to the excessive force of blood coursing through the artery.

* **Alcohol abuse** is toxic to the heart and nervous system.

Risk Factors for Cardiovascular Disease

GENETIC & MEDICAL

-Strong family history of cardiovascular disease (parents, siblings) especially before age sixty.
-Diabetes Mellitus.
-Elevated cholesterol.
-Elevated triglycerides.
-Use of oral contraceptives past the age thirty-five.
-Elevated blood pressure.

LIFESTYLE

-Cigarette smoking.
-Diet high in fat.
-Obesity.
-Chronic stress is now being researched.

Finally, but most importantly for our purposes, is . . .
LACK OF EXERCISE. A sedentary lifestyle contributes to increased cholesterol levels, decreased circulation, obesity and too much risk!

You can take control of heart disease risk factors. Here are some suggestions.

FITNESS OPTIONS

-Cardiorespiratory exercise:
- Increases HDL, promotes less clotting of the blood.
- Lowers level of fat in blood.
- Reduces weight.
- Heart muscle gets stronger, beats slower and increases the volume of blood throughout the body.
- Increase endurance and physical energy.
- Helps lower blood pressure.
- Helps control diabetes.
- Decreases overall stress.

LIFESTYLE OPTIONS

- Low fat diet.
- Reduce alcohol consumption.
- Reduce sodium.
- Do not smoke.
-Participation in stress reduction class, yoga, Tai Chi, meditation, relaxation.
- Support group interaction.

"Use it or lose it."

MASTERS & JOHNSON,
Sex Researchers

CHAPTER 6

Sex

Dateline: May 1995
Leora's Living Room
San Francisco, California

The television is on, but my attention has left the screen due to those lengthy commercial "pauses." I try to ignore the product pushes, but I guess the messages get through to me, because I often find myself singing along word-for-word or repeating the script. Before menopause (BM), I never paid any attention to those adult disposable diaper commercials. Then, I was always baffled–why do they need such a frequent ad? More importantly, why is that famous actress so pleased to have found such a "great, dependable product"? I would have flashbacks to my nursing days circa 1965–working in the geriatric ward and dealing with seventy year old patient's incontinence. BM, I just couldn't figure out those adult diaper commercials because the "patients" didn't look that old!

When I was writing this chapter on sex, including **genital and urinary functions**, one of my clients admitted to me that she uses that "great, dependable product"! At the age of fifty, she suffers from urinary incontinence when she sneezes or laughs and thought there just was nothing to be done about the condition. This is the aspect of menopause and aging that just blows me away! Turns out there are reports that adult disposable diapers outsell the baby version! There are fitness and lifestyle solutions to menopausal conditions regarding sexual, genital and urinary issues. Don't let the advertisements baffle you as they did me!

Urinary Changes

The pelvic floor and abdominal muscles weaken as we age. We may find ourselves getting up frequently through the night to urinate. The loss of muscle tone can lead to "stress incontinence," the tendency to leak urine when you do a sudden movement–like sneezing, coughing, laughing, or sometimes even during movements of exercise–when pressure is put on the bladder. If you are experiencing low abdominal pain or continual need to urinate, see your physician.

Fitness Options

-Lose weight. Extra fat in abdomen puts stress on bladder
-Strengthen abdominal muscles.
    (See exercises in Part Three for details.)
-Do daily Kegels (See description page 82.)

Lifestyle Options

- Go to the bathroom at first urge to urinate.
- Watch diet: spicy foods, alcohol and caffeine can cause
    bladder irritation.

Sexual and Genital Changes

A brand new experience comes with the end of menstruation–not having to worry about birth control and the fear of unplanned pregnancy. Usually at this time, when children grown or close to leaving, living in the "empty nest" would seem to be very liberating for our sex life. However, a frequent complaint from menopausal women is vaginal dryness. This menopausal symptom is one of the frequent reasons women decide to go on Hormone Replacement Therapy

(HRT). During our menstruating years, the mucosa of the vagina is well lubricated and elastic. The surface is thick with many folds of tissue and numerous layers of cells. With the decrease of estrogen, the vagina loses its elasticity and lubricating abilities. The walls become very thin. This is called vaginal atrophy. It can develop anywhere from four to five years after menopause. Sexual arousal causes reduced amount of lubrication and the capacity for vaginal expansion may decrease. This contributes to painful intercourse. It's important at this time to discuss this with your partner as it may be interpreted as disinterest or dislike in sexual relations. Talking may bring about innovative, new approaches to sex making it more exciting . . . perhaps like the early years of your relationship.

An active sex life keeps vagina expanded and prevents atrophy. Masters & Johnson, the sex gurus of the 1970s conducted studies that observed that women who have sex once or twice a week have better and quicker lubrication after menopause. Regular sex increases blood supply to the entire reproductive and urinary area; increases estrogen levels and holds off vaginal atrophy by literally "exercising" the vagina muscles.

Vaginal atrophy is an opportunity to create a renewed sexual experience–the kids are gone, you can't get pregnant, and you are with the person you love! Loving touch such as caressing and massaging improves circulation in the pelvic region. A water soluble lubricant like Astroglide, or Replens, can increase wetness. Do not use oil or petroleum jellies, since there can be an increase of infections of the genital/urinary tract. Estrogen orally or in vaginal creams is effective in treating vaginal atrophy. It is available by prescription from your healthcare provider.

Kegels

Dr. Arnold Kegel developed a special set of exercises in the late 1940s for women to strengthen the PC (pubococcygeal) muscle that helps support the bladder and urethra and the connective tissues that surround the vagina and anus. Women who do these exercises regularly have noticed less leaking of urine on sudden movement, as well as heighten vaginal sensation, including more pleasurable sexual relations. These exercises can be done anywhere–standing, sitting or lying down.

All women should do these exercises during menopause as a preventive measure even if you are not having symptoms.

1. Abdominals and buttocks remain relaxed throughout the exercises.

2. Imagine your pelvic floor as an elevator. Draw up the vaginal muscles one floor at a time, holding three seconds at each floor until you reach floor five. Then relax all muscles. Repeat this process five times.

3. Squeeze your vaginal muscles firmly, hold for three seconds, then relax all. Repeat this process five times.

4. Do "Kegels" daily for optimum results.

PART TWO

The Emotional and Spiritual Issues

"We exist in a rare moment of stability, dependent upon a delicate balance, that could change at any time."

TARTHAN TULKU

CHAPTER 7

Relationships

The R word. Or is it the "Our" Word? Relationships. This is tough stuff anytime, and especially during menopause. This is stuff that we first saw with our parents. This is stuff that we lived through with our brothers and sisters. Then, we have our own family. Sometimes, all we can remember are the "good old days "with our parents and siblings; but we know they were not the "good old days" but we keep comparing, comparing, comparing that which was then, with that which is now. There are so many unconscious "family of origin scenarios" that we lose count and become confused at why we reacted as we did to a perfectly normal situation in "our family."

For example, my "family of origin" was very demonstrative. I was the first-born and the book-worm nerd. So whenever the family was whooping and hollering downstairs, I was upstairs reading. Whenever I was downstairs, they were upstairs, and the eternal question, "Where's Leora?" I was convinced that I certainly was adopted to this wild and crazy family. I always sought escape from the noise. Now, as my husband Dennis sits calmly reading the paper, I am antsy because he's so quiet! I often think, where is the excitement, the noise I cannot escape, and I get angry when he won't leave that newspaper and TALK TO ME! Such is the mysterious overflow from the family we once endured and to whom we are now endeared.

When you really stop to think about it, all our relationships are perfect. Why? Because they teach us balance, a polarity and a lesson due if we are willing to learn. What happens when we as women physically go through menopause while our husbands just age? Our menopause has that physical definition of "end of menstruation" and brings the possibility of new beginnings.

For males, mid-life passages are not so distinct. Men do not experience the sudden decrease in production of sex hormones, but they do experience a mid-life crisis which usually has a psychological basis. The research on male menopause is approximately twenty years behind the study of female menopause (one of the few studies that we as women have the privilege of being first and foremost)! However, some researchers have identified a male menopause referred to as *andropause.* Andropause refers to the gradual decrease in male hormones (androgens). It is indicated to manifest about age sixty, and the symptoms include difficulty maintaining erections, hot flashes, increase in tiredness and sleep disturbances.

Menopause is a subject that men are not very comfortable with. For one primary reason, your menopause is reminder that he, too, is aging. Our menopause has forced us to change. Men do not have such a clear catalyst. Men may experience graying hair or a balding head, a paunchy stomach and muscle aches or pains, but their symptoms are not as pronounced as those experienced by women. Nonetheless, the famous male mid-life crisis rears its ugly head since this is a time when males have concerns about their ability to function sexually, physically, emotionally.

Our menopause gives us a tremendous opportunity to open up a dialogue with our partners about "the change" and explore ways in which we can "change" together. First, we need to look at our relationship with ourselves. We must think–what really is going on with my life–making this a time of introspection and awareness–a time of looking inside and a very personal examination. Am I happy with my career? What about that new career that satisfies your talents and heart? Can I take time to slow down and smell the roses? What about that college degree you were so close to? We now question our life, our career, our being. We wish to savor every present moment, even though sometimes it is baffling, new and strange. Think of this–did you ever imagine you could start all over again at the big 5-0 and create a new YOU? Isn't it exciting to be another person in your body–with options for the future and a strong will to bring your goals to reality? Be a change master!

Having evaluated our relationship with ourselves, now it is time to re-evaluate our primary relationships with our loved ones. Force yourself to take a good look at that person you have spent years with–and recognize that they are looking at you with some of the same thoughts, doubts, and fears. A "how-to-live with-you-now" manual is not available, so it is your responsibility to acquaint your husband and family with this woman who is on the other edge of womanhood. Your body transformation insists upon your emotional transformation. Get comfortable with it and then tell your family about it. This will help you to validate this menopause transition because it has happened and you will never be that person that was present before–at least not entirely. Your entire way of living each day has changed. Acknowledge this, because if you do not, it will annoy you until you do. Accept this person who has emerged out of living through menopause and be willing to freely share your new relationship with you with all your other relationships.

How About Those Mood Swings?

During this time of change in our lives, no doubt you will be the recipient of remarks like "Gosh, you're moody today!" "What's gotten into you?" "Why are you so upset about that?" "Why on earth are you crying now?" It may be helpful to remind your relations, and for you to remember, that you are like an adolescent with your hormones running

amok, dealing with peer pressure to be attractive and popular, all the while trying to figure out what you want to be
when you grow up beyond menopause! So resembling the
stage of puberty, our menopausal moods are affected by the
decrease and fluctuation of hormones in our system as well
as the changes in our lives–children leaving (empty nest syndrome), husband experiencing job change or mid-life issues,
and strained relationships. This is a time of more than just
"our change" and many times, several changes happen at
once, which may lead to anxiety, nervousness and depression.

Mood swings can also can be caused by not getting enough
sleep or insomnia. My ability to sleep through a four alarm
fire changed dramatically after menopause. A formerly heavy
sleeper, I never awakened during the night. During my transition, I fell asleep quickly and then found myself getting up
several times during the night, after tossing and throwing
off the covers. Although I was forty-five years old when this
began, sleeping changes as well as occasional hot flashes can
begin in your thirties, as you approach menopause. These
changes affect us all differently. If losing sleep causes you to
lose your ability to concentrate, are fatigued and irritable–
you, like me, are not a very happy camper.

Several factors are considered responsible for the change in
sleeping pattern:

1) The discomfort of having a night sweat–heat and perspiration is what wakes you up.
2) The hypothalamus, the seat of the sleep center, is specu-
lated to contain estrogen receptors, which decrease in stimulation as estrogen production decreases during menopause.
Hence, less sleep.
3) Our nervous system that controls the "fight or flight"
pattern may become overactive with the shift in body
chemistry, causing an "instant" mood swing to tears.

The good news is that exercise stimulates norepinephrine release in the brain that stabilizes the nervous system. Studies indicate that often when you have suffered from premenstrual syndrome (PMS), symptoms of menopause may be more intense or prolonged. Other research studies have found that the "empty nest" is a welcome relief and the cessation of menstruation for many women is a positive experience.

Mid-life may be a time when women "feel" invisible to men. Remember when they opened the door, gave a lingering look as you passed, were the first to begin the conversation? As we age, the interaction does change, and for women who consciously or unconsciously used their "looks" to operate in the world, this new scenario can be quite scary and another reason for mood swings. As she adjusts to her new MO in life, we see a new emergence of women "hanging out" together at this time. When we are young, we spend time with our girlfriends, as we mature we find ourselves family-centered, spending time with that significant other, and now we find ourselves with our women friends again in a renewed sisterhood brought about by the changes that only we as women are experiencing in our lives and bodies.

To support your relationship with yourself and with others, hanging out with other women in menopause is not such a bad idea. Strong sisterhoods are springing up worldwide in shapes of support groups. (A list is available at the end of this chapter.) From the initial workshops I conducted at Pacific Athletic Club in San Francisco, many women wanted to continue the dialogue that we started. On April 20, 1995, I gave birth to "Mid-life & Beyond", an informational support group based in fitness centers. This group savors the time spent together sharing "women's stories" with nuggets like . . .

"Yippee, it's over!"
"I miss my periods. They were part of my life. A regular cycle."
"What's the big deal. One day it stops."

"I went to buy a book on menopause and placed my credit card over the word."
"When I went to find herbal remedies, I asked for the PMS section."
"I feel old."
"No more PMS!"
"No more birth control!"

Here's a story that I shared recently about empowerment. When I was young, everyone called me Lee. Part of this was my reluctance, my shyness, my timidity to correct them when they mispronounced my name–Lorna, Leonara, Lenora, Leroy etc . . . I will never forget the day (sometime around age twenty) that I corrected someone's pronunciation of my name. My self-esteem enabled me to be assertive and insist that that person pronounce my name correctly. It was a wonderful feeling of empowerment. I get that same sensation every time I speak my mind today. I am not worried about the consequences, I just want to make sure that you know what I mean. Not a negative, just a straight forward declaration! Like writing this book–putting these thoughts on paper to share with someone who cares, like you!

One of my great joys in working with body-based approaches to health and wellness is the appreciation of actual proof of change. I am aware of all the changes that my clients make–exercise, nutrition, lifestyle and fitness–they all have a measurable effect, which in turn motivates them to continue. You can experience this, too! Physical change creates motivation that creates continual successes every time you exercise. Many clients come to me that have never completed anything in their life. Every time they complete a training session they have achieved success at completion that carries over to other life activities. The body will reflect measurable change–that is the indicator that proves that you have the power to change some-thing, any-thing, in your life.

So what I am saying is STRUT YOUR STUFF!! With the knowledge (which you have after reading this book) comes power. Choose to make menopause a new life adventure and please, break the news to your relations, your family. Let them in on your new vision of you and how they, your primary relationships, can help you embrace the future of living beyond menopause.

Here's some ideas to smooth those relationships and make those mood swings and insomnia a bit less severe.

FITNESS OPTIONS

-Regular exercise gives a sense of accomplishment (success) as well as sense of well-being from the endorphins in the system. Exercise releases endorphins that have analgesic effect and give sense of well- being.
-Exercise, when completed, is an instant success and accomplishment.
-Exercise on a regular basis increases ability to sleep. If you are an early morning exerciser, change schedule. A late afternoon workout may be a better option if you are having difficulty sleeping.
-Create a workout, challenging mind and body like martial arts, dance, wall climbing, archery, yoga, stretch relaxation class, and Tai Chi to release tension and balance moodiness.
-Do not perform vigorous exercise close to the time you retire.
-Stretching exercises release muscular tension and calms the body and spirit.

LIFESTYLE OPTIONS

-Reduce coffee and sugar—both are stimulants creating ups and downs in your moods.
-Avoid coffee after 12 Noon.
-Avoid alcohol at least four hours before going to bed.

-Keep room cool and sleep in light clothes and bed
   coverings.
-Take a hot bath before going to bed. Add Kneipp®, or
   other relaxing herbs to bath water to soothe and
   harmonize yourself.
-If awakened and you cannot get back to sleep, take a
   warm shower or bath, and have a banana or cereal
   with low-fat milk.
-Inquire about Hormone Replacement Therapy (HRT)
   to alleviate dramatic mood swings and insomnia
   symptoms.

Menopause Support Groups

*For a guide for organizing your own
support group, contact:*

American Self-Help Clearinghouse
Attn.: Menopause How-To
St. Clare's-Riverside Medical Center
25 Pocono Road
Denville, New Jersey 07834
Phone: (201) 625-7101

North American Menopause Society
C/O Cleveland Medical Clinic
29001 Cedar Road #600
Cleveland, Ohio 44124
Phone: (216) 844-3334

Mid-Life & Beyond
A Fitness Based Support Group
4338 California Street
San Francisco, CA 94118
(415) 221-2683
Leora Myers, R.N., Founder

"Even a tarnished mirror will shine like a jewel if it is polished. A mind which is presently closed by illusions originating from the innate darkness of life is like a tarnished mirror, but once it is polished it will become clear, reflecting the enlighten- ment of immutable truth."

NICHIREN DAISHONIN
Major Writings of Nichiren Daishonin, Volume I

CHAPTER 8

Spiritual Transformation

When I look at the words "spiritual transformation," I am not talking about religion. I am talking about what makes you–who you are. My definition of "spiritual" is an awareness of one's spirit, of one's self–of that which makes us who we are. I believe that menopause gives us a chance to take a spiritual pause and reflect and identify even more closely with our spiritual nature. I cannot define what is spiritual for you, but I want to share with you my spiritual transformation story and maybe awaken your own process.

One morning when I was sixteen years old, I sat straight up in the bed with a very clear message echoing loudly in my brain–I am going to be a nun! I ceremoniously brushed my teeth, got dressed, all done-up with a new feeling consuming me–Leora, you have had a vision of what your mission in life is–you will enter the convent and become a nun. I floated down the stairs for breakfast and everyone in my family appeared different to me–like having been chosen, my family will have a nun for a sister and daughter. I ate differently, carefully placing the food in my mouth as a nun would. I felt totally different, as I knew in my heart, and really felt, that I would be a fine nun. I am not sure how long this feeling lasted, perhaps a few months. Yet, as quickly as it came, it went. It just seemed to fall out of my body and consciousness.

My family were devout Catholics–saying the Rosary every night and attending Mass every Sunday. I enjoyed the ceremonies and the mysterious Latin language. I even took Latin I & II in high school. Since I attended Catholic grammar school and college, the nuns were my curriculum mentors as well as very good business women. I do owe my tenacity to them, and the realization that there are rewards if you are financially successful–like no homework if you sell the most candy bars!

In college courses I became a Catholic rebel, particularly in Father Murphy's Theology class–always fertile ground for challenge. I just wanted to know why, if God loved all of us, what about the millions of people who are good and honest but not Catholic–what will happen to all of them when they die? I recently looked at my grades from college, and I understand why I received all "A" and "B" grades except for Father Murphy's "C "and "C-" ratings! I had always thought of myself as a spiritual, as opposed to a religious person. Now I see why I was so emphatic about how envisioned myself.

When I graduated from college and began my nursing career, my occasions at Mass were sporadic. I always felt a special solitude and peace when I was inside the church, yet it left me at the doorstep when I left the building. I felt a Catholic education was the best, so my son Michael went to St. Dominic's Grammar School and Sacred Heart High School. Plus, let's face it, they had the best basketball teams! Michael succeeded in being named to the All State High School team and was honored as "Most Inspirational" which made me very proud.

My move to California was the catalyst and the place for my spiritual transformation. Believe me, I dabbled in every course to find my spirit–EST, psychic readings, tarot, numerology, visualization. My own business, Creative Bodywork Center, hosted many workshops on these subjects, but I came to the conclusion that our name really did suggest body-based programs. That was my first transformation and I decided to go mainstream. I got rid of the earth shoes and the natural hair-do (my parents were so thrilled) and began consulting with corporations because I was (and I am) convinced that these people need bodywork and fitness, too.

As I embarked on providing classes for major corporations like Levi Strauss & Co, Apple, IBM, and Lockheed, one essence always came through in my work. Clients would tell me "I feel so uplifted after your class", "I always feel you touch something inside me with your class, a feeling I don't feel in other classes." Although I was "mainstream," in corporate settings, my essence, my spirit, is what touched people, along with fitness programs that gave them results.

With my success intact, I still sensed there was something missing. Just like my logo–all bodies balanced–my body was great, my emotional self felt flexible, strong and centered, yet I felt my spiritual body needed a daily practice just as much as my physical body. This feeling came at a time that many of us start questioning–I was 44 years old. We know what we are capable of producing in our work, careers, and relationships, yet we also wish to find what our spirit is–how it affects our life and what it is capable of experiencing. The questions of who are we, what are we meant to do, to be and what is true happiness for this spirit? They all started to dominate me.

As a young child, I had always been intrigued with Japan. I found an oriental robe and every Halloween, I dressed as a Japanese woman, until one year, I could not find it. My Mother confessed years later that she had hidden it, because she was so sick of seeing that robe every year. Also, there was a ceramic bowl on Grandmother Marie's cocktail table that fascinated me. Repeatedly, I was told not to touch it, until finally, my long-suffering relatives found it more practical just to put it away when I came to visit. I have that bowl now! It is a painting of Buddha in front of Mount Fuji. I also number-painted a Japanese woman in front of a Buddha statue when I was sixteen. As we come to realize, nothing is an accident in life.

In the early 1980's, I read Tina Turner's book, *I, TINA*, and I have never forgotten how Tina said that her life turned around when she began chanting and became a Buddhist. Her story of overcoming challenges and revitalizing her life through a spiritual change made an indelible impression on me. A clear, resonant, inner voice said to me–I want to do that. A couple of years passed, and I saw an article about Tina in a magazine, complete with a picture of her chanting in front of her Buddhist altar. The same clear, resonant but even louder voice said to me again–I want to do that. Years passed, until one day, I attended a workshop with Raul Espinoza, a colleague I had known for quite some time. He seemed to be a different person than the one I knew before– formerly a frantic, anxious person, now, he seemed relaxed, centered and very comfortable to be with. He told me that he had begun to practice Nichiren Daishonin Buddhism and chanted Nam-Myoho-Renge-Kyo. Those words were the same words that Tina had said in her book.

My inner voice that had said–I want to do that–was finally answered. The next week, my friend took me to meet others that chanted and I began my daily spiritual practice on April 30, 1986, that continues to this day. In 1987, I was fortunate to be invited to be the United States fitness trainer for instructors at the newly opened Nautilus of Japan. There, I was able to visit the main temple which was nestled at the bottom of Mount Fuji, the mountain that was pictured on my grandmother's bowl.

Now, at this change of life, is time–to find time to be with your Self. You are **BODY-MIND-SPIRIT**. With the balance of our self, we uncover our true mission. Believe me–it is not easy like A-B-C–which you may think just by reading this book. Every change I have made has taken a total commitment, and it has not always been easy. In fact, big steps take incredible courage, tenacity and hope. There have been times when I have felt that I just can't do it. In the silence of thought, meditation and contemplation, the solution for me has evolved and I am made aware of why all the situations that came before were necessary in the BIG PLAN.

My mission on menopause and beyond has arisen out of my spiritual transformation. At one time, I thought I would be the QUEEN OF AEROBICS, the next JANE FONDA, the OPRAH WINFREY OF FITNESS. Well, if anyone had told me that I would conduct worldwide workshops on menopause and publish a book on menopause, I would have said you are out of your mind! It's no accident–this is what I am supposed to do. It was no accident that I am a registered nurse and have spent years combining fitness and health consulting, had a challenging menopause, and added the spiritual component to my life. These were all important events in the course of finding my true mission in life.

Please don't negate your own life experiences. They are all important when you look at the big picture. You do have a way to validate your life experience–what gives you the most joy, when are you most happy–whatever you are doing then is what you are supposed to be doing. If you are not happy, it probably is because it is not what you are supposed to be doing. Mid-life is a time when your options are up to you. Yes, you can return to school. Yes, you can move into a career that has always been interesting to you and you felt you had an innate talent for it. The element that is keeping you back is YOU!!!!

I tell you this story to characterize my personal journey–to find the link I needed, to find who I really am and how to "polish" my spirit, my inner self, that which makes me Leora– to look clearly into the mirror and see "me." I share this story to encourage you to seek and discover that which makes you who you are. After you find that, continue to practice methods that continually uncover that spiritual part of you. GO FOR IT!

"As a woman experiences her life, it is important for her to name her experiences in words. When one woman puts her experiences into words, another woman who has kept silent, afraid of what others will think, can find validation, and when the second woman says aloud, 'Yes, that was my expierence, too,' the first woman loses some of her fear."

CAROL P. CHRIST
Diving Deep and Surfacing:
Women Writers on Spiritual Quest

CHAPTER 9

Letters from the Heart

When I began conducting my lectures and workshops, my sister Ethel gave me Carol's wonderful quote. She said, "Food for thought to incorporate into your speeches, Leora." How true! In order to deal more effectively with the emotional and spiritual issues that the physical change of menopause inspires, I have found the technique of journalizing my thoughts on paper to be very cleansing. (After all, that's how this book began!) I highly recommend this activity to women in my workshops and classes. There is something so powerful about putting your thoughts, your emotions, your goals, onto paper.

The following six letters reflect the feelings of women who are moving in, through, and beyond menopause. With their complete permission and blessing, I share them with you now, perhaps unlocking your own story, a letter waiting to be written, from your heart . . .

Dear Leora:

When I found out I was pregnant the first time, some four years ago, I knew immediately that I wanted to have my child at home with as little medical intervention as possible. I started to physically train my body with an intensity I had never found necessary before in my life. I did yoga twice a week, aerobics three times a week and I swam at least five times a week. Prior to this I'd been a yo-yo dieter who smoked to keep a girlish figure. The reality of motherhood had already begun to change me physically, spiritually and mentally.

My son Jake is three an a half years old now and I am pregnant again. More than ever I am aware of the importance of a physical fitness regimen for myself. Not only does it keep my body in shape and capable to endure the rigors of work and mothering, but it means I take special time for myself daily . . . I want my lifestyle to be a model to my children. And when my beautiful children are grown and gone, I want my body and my life healthy and strong for me.

Cheryl Madsen
33 years young
Theater Manager
San Francisco, California

June 10, 1995

Dear Leora;
In the past year, at the age of 41, I have reached a level of
physical fitness which I am very happy with. I was
surprised to see the physical changes I could achieve at
my age. Here is a list of benefits of exercising which
includes taking your SuperShaping Class twice a week:
- Feeling well physically
- Feeling strong
- Being proud of the changes with my body
- Gaining trust in myself to be in control of my physical
condition
- Accepting the fact that I deserve to be happy with
myself physically as well as emotionally.
Reaching this level has helped me understand my own
capabilities more and has given me a positive outlook on
my direct effect on my own life. As I move towards my
future and the inevitable changes that will occur with
my body, due to the aging process, I plan to continue
working out to my fullest ability.

Sincerely,
Lori Gfroerer
41 years young
Redwood Shores, California

June 10, 1995

To My Daughter, Mahogany
I am writing you to talk about this passage of time called mid-life. Although it is in the distant future, you too will be sharing this experience, I am 44 years old and feel like I am in the prime of my life. My health is good and the shape and condition of my body is better than ever. Here's why . . . After I began working at the University in 1990, I realized my sedentary lifestyle could not continue. Basically, my only exercise was walking to and from the bus stop or parking lot. My office was located in the same building as the gym so I decided to take a class. I had not exercised since high school so I started with the "stretch & tone" class. It was slow and relaxing but soon I knew I was ready for a bigger challenge. The next class I took was "low impact" and soon graduated to "step aerobics." I fell in love with this class. I went three times a week for two years. (Remembered Dennis bought me a step instead of the tennis bracelet I wanted.) I remembered how I envied this young instructor's muscles. Her arms and back were gorgeous. After the first year we added resistance–hand weights and rubber bands–anything to create resistance and build muscle while stepping. The workout was grueling but it worked. The definition in my back was complemented by a fellow student in class and my thighs had slimmed down to the point I could wear a dress that I had not been able to wear before.

A drawback to Step was lunge movements that injured my heel causing difficulty walking and stopping all exercise for weeks. The instructor had mentioned that she received her certification from Leora Myers, who happened to be a friend of mine. I signed up for Leora's SuperShaping Class which consisted of slow, controlled exercises done with ankle and hand weights. I enjoyed these workouts which required less youthful exuberant energy, less stepping up and down, more focused concentration AND gave me the results I wanted. Watching Leora instruct the class, I saw how she had defined the areas of her body that I too want to change. It was wonderful to see actual proof.

So today, my current routine involves walking home from work every day (2.5 miles) and SuperShaping twice a week. I am sharing all of this with you to encourage you to continue throughout your life with your own exercise program, swimming, basketball, softball and bike riding. I firmly believe that keeping your body fit will increase your stamina, strengthen your heart and prolong your life.

Love,
Mom
A.k.a.
Sylviaette Gamble
46 years young
Program Assistant
Women's Resource Center
San Francisco, California

Dear Me,
The trouble with menopause is that it comes at a bad age.
If we went through menopause at age 20, there would be
no stigma attached to it. I hate it! If one more person
says I look good "for my age," I'm going to have to
punish him or her. To paraphrase Gloria Steinem and
Leora Myers, "This is what 50 looks like!" When my
friend, with whom I lift weights with, had a party to
celebrate the completion of her "change," I wrote her this
little ditty:

Girlfriends.
They're there at puberty.
They're there at maturity.
May they always be there.
For you, and for me.

Cheryl H. Ruby, Ph.D.
51 years young
San Francisco, California

June 3, 1995

To My Friend, Velma
We met on vacation in Maui when our children were
playing with their shovels and pails in the sand. All
those late nights we spent on the beach listening to the
waves and wondering if these kids would ever grow up!
Can you believe the kids are graduating from high
school? Well, they have and so have we. Look at how far
we've come! We're 50 years old and better than ever. I
never thought I'd feel so young when mid-life ap-
proached me. Maybe it's because I'm in better shape
today. I take care of myself. I try to eat 4 fruits and
vegetables a day and drink lots of water, but water has
always been my drink of choice.
Staying in shape has become one of my priorities. Not
only do I play tennis 4 times a week, but I work out, too.
Since I've joined a gym, my body has definitely changed
and I am strong, fit and focused. I feel great. I like the
way I look and feel. Those hot flashes, they don't bother
me. They come & go, but they don't get me down. I have
too many other priorities in my life. Aren't you glad we
live in a time when people care about themselves?

Diane Klein
52 1/2 young
Hillsborough, California

Dear Leora,

Staying fit at 55 years old is more of a challenge than it used to be. While feeling uplifted and emotionally energized after a workout, I often am glad to sit for a while at work and often wish to take a nap. Always having been a very physically active person, my daily exercise regimen is not much different in my 50's than it was in my 30's. I approach exercise with much the same attitude as I do many other things in my life. Being rebellious and curious by nature, I tend to challenge our traditional notions about aging. I suspect most people simply believe what they are told. They give up, get lazy or passive and they become old. I don't believe much of what I'm told without challenging it, so why should I be different about aging!

Ellie Hessl
55 years young
Marriage, Family and Child Counselor,
Hillsborough, California

PART THREE

Leora's Complete Exercise Guide

> *"Our self-image consists of four
> components that are involved in
> every action: movement, sensation,
> feeling and thought."*
>
> MOSHE FELDENKRAIS

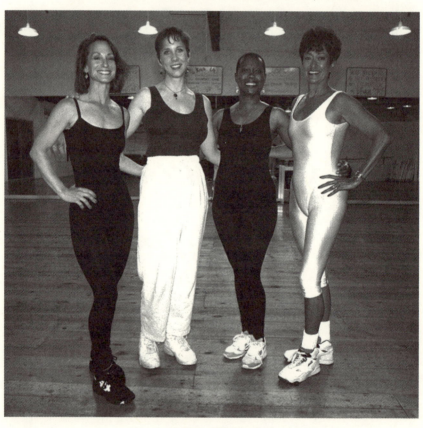

Left to Right:
Exercise Models Lori Gfroerer,
Cheryl Madsen, Sylviaette Gamble,
and Ellie Hessl

CHAPTER 10

Every Picture Tells A Story

REAL WOMEN REALLY DO EXERCISE

The Women

I created my "Fitness Plan For Life" for the bodies, hearts and souls of real people, just like you! I believe that my plan's ability to transform your life can best be illustrated by some of my students. Throughout Part Three, you will find my words supported by the photographed bodies of these fine women–thank you (and all those who were unable to attend our June 10 photo session) from the depths of my heart and soul! These four women are symbolic of the message of this book and I appreciate each one of them for their contribution.

Cheryl Madsen, 33 years young, embracing one of women's greatest arts–bringing life into the world. Three months pregnant and lifting weights; quite a different scenario than during the carrying of Jake, her first pregnancy. Cheryl's contribution portrays the full spectrum of womanhood–reproduction to passage of change. It is a circle. Cheryl, I hope you have a girl, so you can give her this book–a birth to the passage of change guide!

Lori Grfoerer, 41 years young, has astounding ability to change herself. Three years after I began challenging Lori's concentration, focus and willingness to trust my methodology, a new physical and emotional definition evolved, along with renewed awareness of her ability to transform herself as well as others. I see her special talent is as a teacher, ready to share her passage of transformation . . . ready to bloom!

Sylviaette Gamble, 44 years young, is the "Ralph Nader" of fitness programs. The course has to feel right to all her body parts, be cost effective and the instructor has to display "actual proof" of positive effects. I am so glad I passed her tests! She is hanging tough in my classes, looking good and feeling stronger than she has ever imagined. Although Sylviaette did not begin exercising until she was forty, she is a firm believer that fitness is the way to a long, healthy life.

Ellie Hessl, 55 year young, is a great player in this endeavor. She gave me information about the first menopause workshop I ever attended. There, I met Dr. Sadja Greenwood, who told me to write this book. I am always impressed with Ellie's determination to stay strong and healthy for a long, long time as well as her willingness to learn new methodology to enhance the quality of her life–today and tomorrow.

Real Women Demand A Real Plan

My logo, designed by Paul Kagawa, pictured above, possesses three bodies–symbolizing **"We are One: Body-Mind-Spirit."** The circle represents unending determination; whereas the triangle, which is inverted, symbolizes the female aspect of the pyramid. In 1975, my first vision, the Creative Bodywork Center, became a reality. All the experiences that had transformed *my body* and *my awareness* were now classes offered at the Center: yoga, Tai Chi, massage and dance exercise, as well as weekend seminars on relaxation, massage techniques–shiatsu, accupressure, Esalen, Feldenkrais, Rolfing and creative visualization. My Center was considered strange and way-out back then. I find it interesting that twenty years later, we see these same programs emerging in health centers, hospitals and corporations as valuable components for enhancing the quality of life.

My early involvement in my business included just about everything: developing the curriculum, selecting the best teachers and registering the students. The other time was spent extending my own "body sabbatical." I took classes at my Center as well as continued studying dance. San Francisco had a wealth of incredible teachers and I had the fortune to study with the best–jazz with Ed Mock; Katherine Dunham technique with Ruth Beckford (Miss B.); African dance with Raymond Sawyer and Malonga Casquelord and ballet at the San Francisco Dance Studio. My mother Adelaide, who often visited, shared my enthusiasm and came to watch classes. I remember her surprise that I would quite literally follow in her dance steps.

 The most popular class at the my Center (the one that helped pay the rent) was a dance exercise class–that was the title we used before "aerobics." My instructor, Helene Zynstein, was offered an opportunity to teach at another private facility. She gave me her two weeks notice and notified her loyal students that she was leaving. "Either you find us a great teacher or we're out of here!!" were my greetings from Helene's students. Luckily, I'm good at adversity! I knew that I would have to keep these ladies, since it was my most popular class (and it helped pay the rent). I figured that I've taken Helene's class, I know her format–maybe I'll fill in until I find a replacement. So, I took the next two weeks to develop a class, practicing day and night. I pulled the elements and strengths from all my disciplines to develop my first "dance exercise" class–transcultural movements and music, yoga stretches, visualization at the beginning as well as the task maker's demand for excellence and 100 percent effort in every move–an excellence I learned in the hours spent with my movement masters–Beckford, Mock, Sawyer and Masquelord. I chose to end my version of Helene's class with relaxation and Tai Chi.

The first day I taught, I walked into my exercise room, put my music on (records back then), took a deep breath, faced the ladies, who had a "show me" look on their faces, and began. At the end of class, they roared and applauded and yelled," It's THE BEST WORKOUT IN TOWN!!!!" That phrase became my trademark, the name of my class, and I ended up expanding to additional classes at my Center, as well as conducting a Sunday class accompanied by live, percussion music–again, a first in the fitness industry. Strange and way-out in the 1970s, today, it is considered innovative and creative with worldwide requests! I even directed classes at Levi Strauss' fitness center, one of the first corporate-based fitness facilities. I trained instructors and my bodysculpting system, SuperShaping™, expanded to the fitness facilities of IBM, Apple and Lockheed.

Since I couldn't clone myself, I developed a program to train other instructors in the methodology that had made my classes successful–one that included all the elements that made my work successful–scientific, medical knowledge of the body as well as the integration of strength, endurance, flexibility and motivation by constant physical and mental challenge for all participants. Today, my schedule includes personal fitness training in clients' homes and gyms, teaching SuperShaping™ and traveling throughout the word lecturing, conducting seminars and taking Fitness holidays where my clients join me for a spa vacation.

The future: my own spa retreat on an island in Greece where women come together to re-new, re-juvenate and re-ignite their physical, emotional, spiritual self. A place of safe passage. You are invited to join me there in the new millennium!

Right now, it's time for you to get FIT! But why? If you are committed to exercise, you probably know the answer, but have not put it in words. If you have slackened or quit your exercise program, you know there is something missing in life. Here's the answer: WE, who are committed to a regular exercise program, continue to exercise for the immediate feeling experienced on accomplishment of the exercise. Without a doubt, every time you exercise, you feel better at completion. So, people exercise for the effect it has on how they feel immediately after completion. It is a predictable result. I tell my clients, "Just walk in that door, you will feel renewed and refreshed at the end of the session"–regardless of what personal problems are facing you–money, relationships, career et al . . .

Of course, physical changes such as reduced body fat, increased strength and tone, and increased flexibility are goals, too, but what keeps us exercising on a regular basis is this fact. Regardless of what is going on in our life, we feel better after that exercise session–every single time! So the concept of body-mind-spirit should be easier to grasp now. There is a definite effect on our mind and spirit when we physically challenge our bodies.

Body-based approaches to well-being–this is my nursing specialty–using the body as basis for changing our lives. We often assume changes have occurred–my relationships are better; I am a more responsible person than I used to be–yet in reality, we are handling things the same way! Working with the body gives you actual proof of the change–that can be measured and physically felt. For example–my clothes size has changed, I wear clothes I couldn't fit into before; I can do twelve straight leg push ups and I started with two on my knees; I can hike five miles easily and last year one mile was my limit; I now ski all day with strength and energy plus I'm not sore.

When you commit to that workout, that class, that training– you choose to overcome all the stresses put to you. At the end, you have a sense of accomplishment and completion. YOU HAVE AN IMMEDIATE SUCCESS. Every time you exercise, you choose to undertake the task, to go through the challenges and stay to the end-point–the accomplishment, the win!

Now, don't you think repeated behavior like this carries over into daily life? You had better believe it! You can see the true meaning about exercise reducing stress–not only at the moment you are exercising, but also when you are asked to take on more stress than you are accustomed to–job/career, home, life, relationships–your physical training has given you training in facing the obstacle, going through the challenge and having success and completion of your goal.

Many of my students have never pushed to the last repetition (in anything) like I demand. However, when they trust my methodology, begin to feel and see results, they begin to trust their own ability to change their lives. This is why I treasure my work–body based approaches to well-being. Working with a real body, a constant source of change–I can measure it, feel it, weigh it, see it. I am capable of effecting change physically therefore I am capable of effecting change in my life.

STRONG BODY=FLEXIBLE MIND=TOUGH SPIRIT

Leora's Fitness Methodology

Foremost, the effectiveness of an exercise program is determined by the execution of every movement. Have you ever seen a person who works out for hours a day and their body never changes compared to the person that works out two-to-three times a week for forty-five minutes to an hour and makes dramatic changes in tone and shape? The difference? The execution of movement. Each movement is important! If you want to develop maximal benefit in the least amount of time and in the safest manner, the form in which an exercise is executed is of most importance. An ideal way to insure form and alignment is to invest in a personal fitness trainer to supervise your workout for important feedback.

My instructing methodology for exercise programs consist of three progressions.

1. Explanation and Demonstration

The first time an exercise is taught, I explain the muscle, the proper form and execution and make immediate corrections so the brain and muscle assimilate the correct information. The form that is executed first is the one that remains in body and mind. We all know how difficult it is to fine tune a tennis or golf game after years of playing the same, old way.

2. Reinforcement

Once learned and repeated correctly, I reinforce the positive execution of movement and make necessary corrections. The student is now in the "groove" of mastered execution and I now begin to demand more–reps, and weight as well as less time between sets.

3. The Push

The repetitions and weight are now at the maximum so that proper form and execution can remain intact. The body has now adapted to this routine and is able to execute each exercise without any danger of injury. I now push through the mental aspect of training. I become the drill sergeant, demanding perfect execution with each repetition, complete mental concentration and undivided focus to the task at hand, with very little rest between sets and exercises.

Result: the body has now adapted and it is time for a new format of exercises.

The body is always trying to adapt to the program it is given. While it is adapting, it is changing as it tries to figures out your plan. Your body changes physically as it adapts. Your body is always changing, let's face it–but when you exercise, you determine the change and can make it a positive change. In my SuperShaping™, this process happens within a six week format. With my Personal Fitness Training clients, this process is developed by adding new machines, exercises, poundage and challenges.

My methodology is based on the way we learn exercise. It takes time for the brain to coordinate the desired skill with the body. Neuromuscular change comes first, followed by skilled execution and then adaptation. Hopefully, this information demonstrates the possibilities for designing your program with consistent challenge:

First: Learn completely the form and execution of all exercises. Take the time.

Second: Feel confident about your execution and push forward.

Third: Challenge your workout by adding poundage, difficulty of exercise, shortened rest between sets and MAINTAIN EXCELLENT FORM ALWAYS.

Fourth: let that routine go and start again on another.

Challenge yourself with this format, making each workout progressive, challenging and ever-changing.

Leora's Fitness Techniques

1. Full Range of Movement

"Straighten your arms," I shout to new students as they do bicep curls. For example, why don't they straighten their arms at the end of a movement? Because it is easier not to. More reps can be accomplished from bent arms than straight. "Every rep counts! Start from a fresh start each rep," I say. "But its harder that way," students say. And I reply, "That's the name of this game–make the exercise more difficult–that is how you get stronger!" Full range of movement insures your muscles are strengthened through their full range of motion, including the weakest position–stretched. This also allows for muscles to be maximally developed.

2. Speed of Movement

Lifting or raising a weight is only half of the exercise. Lowering the weight is the other half. Most people think lifting is work, and lowering is rest, which usually turns into dropping the weight. Lifting is referred to as the positive or concentric phase (shortening of the muscle) and lowering is referred to as the negative or eccentric phase (lengthening of the muscle). The same muscle is used for each phase. As the weight is lowered, the muscles are stretched and prepare for the next contraction. By lowering the weight slowly, you take advantage of getting stronger using the second half of the contraction; decreasing injury which usually occurs when the weight is dropped, and increasing flexibility going through full range of movement

A typical count to work both the concentric and eccentric phases of a contraction is–raise or lift the weight in two counts, pause at full contraction for two counts and lower in four counts. Do not hold the breath in the pause at full contraction. When using weight, by not allowing the plates to rest on the weight stack, or dropping a weighted body part to floor in an exercise class, muscle tension is maintained through the exercise set.

3. Warm-up
A conscious awareness that you are about to exercise. It is a transition that says you are about to leave other activities in your day and engage mentally and physically in the task at hand. The warm-up is a "beginning" ritual that will automatically signal to your body that this is its time to exercise. Have a definite beginning. If you are working out at home, insure there no are distractions–put the answering machine on and volume down so you are not tempted to pick up that one call; family and friends at home know to "do not disturb"; allot enough time for an unhurried workout and have a definite stretch or movement that signifies this beginning. In class, we take a deep breath and stretch up. My clients warm up on the treadmill until I come "retrieve" them. Some rituals are unconscious ones. I have seen plenty of joggers pull up their socks and look at their watch before they set off. Whatever, it is a ritual that says to your body–it is time to exercise!

4. Physical Warm-up
Now, we get can get physical and begin a slow, rhythmic exercise of large muscle groups done before an activity. It elevates your body's core temperature and heart rate, as well as increases the blood flow and oxygen to the muscles you will be using in your workout. It is a graduated movement utilizing large muscles in a controlled, full range of motion. A typical warm up last five to ten minutes.

5. Mental Warm-up.

As you physically warm up, mentally think of the workout before you–create vivid mental images of your self as you want to be–strong, flexible, motivated, easily accomplishing each exercise. See the results beginning to happen with each exercise you carry out.

6. Cool-down

This is a conscious awareness that you have completed your workout. It also is a transition signal of completion to your body. Again, do not allow disturbances in this important part of your workout–phone off, do not disturb on, no appointments scheduled right after the end of your exercise session. Have a definite ending. It can be a short relaxation followed by a stretch, it can just be a stretch. I have a movement that ends all my classes. It is my students' symbol of completion–four stretches upward, stretch each arm to the side then down, ending with circling arms upward as we take in a deep breath and release with the arms down to the side. Having a ritual says–I am satisfied, I have completed my exercise.

7. Physical Cool-down

It is the reverse action of the warm up and a gradual *decrease* in exercise intensity using large muscles groups in a controlled manner. It prevents the sudden pooling of blood in the veins, prevents delayed muscle stiffness and soreness, as well as reduces any tendency toward post-exercise stiffness of dizziness. Cool-down also lowers the probability of post-exercise disturbances in the cardiac rhythm. A typical cool down should last five to ten minutes.

8. Mental Cool-down

As you physically cool down, turn your thoughts to winding down from a great workout. Mentally retrace the workout you have just accomplished with a sense of victory. You took action to meet your goals!

The cool down signals the end of that part of your day and releases your mind and body to move on–with the benefits of the workout, increased stamina, feeling of well-being.

9. Mindful Execution

Bring your full awareness to the body part you are working.

Create stabilization that supports your entire body, enabling you to devote full attention to the present exercise. As you move through the exercise, feel the movement, visualize the results and be at full attention to the movement.

10. Challenge Your Body

A muscle will gain strength when it is fully challenged. Less demand than you are capable of handling yields less improvement. This is this purpose of increasing weight, shortening time between sets and adding more difficult exercises.

11. Variety

Machine weights, free weights, body weight. Sequence of exercises. Different exercises. Keeping the body at alert. Never letting it adapt and figure things out. Always giving yourself a new challenge. The spice of life!

12. Starting Position

This is the pre-stretch position where each rep should begin, ALWAYS.

13. Neutral Alignment

Remember when we were told to always do a pelvic tilt and flatten our backs to the floor while doing abdominals? Research now indicates that neutral alignment is preferable in all movements for injury prevention and effectiveness of exercise. Also referred to as neutral spine, this guideline refers to maintaining the natural curves of the back. To find your neutral alignment, lie on floor with knees bent and feet flat on floor, slowly begin to extend your back (arch) slightly and then flex (round) slightly. Continue until you find the position that feels best to your back–that is your neutral spine while lying. Now, sit in a chair with feet planted on floor. Slowly extend and slowly flex your spine until you come to the most comfortable, pain-free position. This is your neutral spine sitting. Now stand and repeat the exercise. This is your standing neutral spine. It is a position of stability–if someone pushed on your shoulder, you would not budge. Experiment with all these techniques. Keep this neutral alignment in all exercises and daily while at work, standing in line at grocery store, or driving your car. It insures safe execution and efficiency of movement as well as increases your energy level throughout the day.

Leora's Real Body As An Anatomy Chart

"Who said this section is about your personal body? We just want to see real women, not stick figures, showing muscle groups and doing exercises!" My editor Laura exclaimed as we discussed this part, and I wailed "But, I'm not ready to be photographed!" Out of resistance comes these reference photos. May you see that fitness can be a way of life for EVERY BODY . . . preparing for, going through and after menopause.

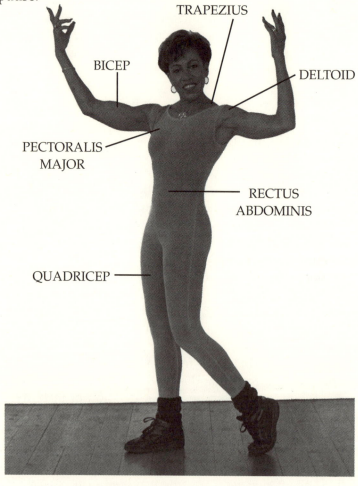

ANTERIOR VIEW OF MUSCLES

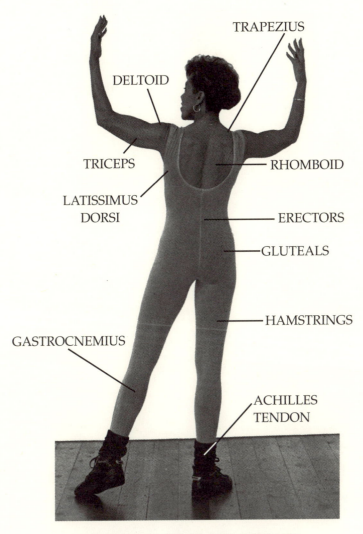

TRAPEZIUS

DELTOID

TRICEPS

RHOMBOID

LATISSIMUS
DORSI

ERECTORS

GLUTEALS

HAMSTRINGS

GASTROCNEMIUS

ACHILLES
TENDON

POSTERIOR VIEW OF MUSCLES

123

"Considering change does one of two things: it either reinforces the rightness of the current situation, or it allows one to find something better."

ANONYMOUS

CHAPTER 11

Weight Training

(BUT I DON'T WANT TO LOOK LIKE ARNOLD!)

Dateline: August 1976
Moss Beach, California

"CLANG CLANG CLANG" was a frequent interruption to the soothing sound of the ocean waves that lapped against our home at the water's edge in this small coastal town. Early evening was a special time for our family; except when I had to listen to the menacing sounds of my husband Dennis lifting weights for hours in a room downstairs. "CLANG CLANG CLANG" went the barbells. (No wonder they call them bar BELLS!) He repeatedly invited me to join him, but I snubbed my nose at such a barbaric form of exercise. "I do AEROBICS," I would say, with the attitude that weight lifting is beneath me. Furthermore, I never wanted those unsightly, bulging muscles. Dennis spent so much time in his gym that I began to regard this activity as "the other woman," whom I jokingly named "Gymallia."

Finally, wanting to spend some more time with Dennis, I descended into the world of iron. The rush I got after completing my first bench press was a sensation I had never felt in any aerobics class. The interaction with the weight was one of challenge. The desire to win the battle of that last repetition was new to this Minnesotan, who grew up avoiding any activity that involved aggression or sweat. It was different from the long endurance dance of aerobics . . . it was a "challenge and rest rhythm."

Five years later, in a hot, steamy arena in Fairfield, California (1981), I am pleased to report that the following announcement occurred: "In second place of the middle weight women's body building competition is Leora Myers."

Tight, lean muscles. In those early years, I felt so many pairs of eyes watching the transformation of my body–displaying changes that only strength work can produce. I felt the stares of my long-term students who resisted the idea of pumping iron, but were intrigued and impressed with the definition and tone that improved week by week. Their bodies were challenged with tougher classes as their teacher got stronger. Newcomers to my studio were not as enthralled with the "tight, lean look" and the word spread, "I'm not working out with her. She's got muscles!" Remember, this was 1981. Muscular women just were not fashionable.

As I got closer to the competition, my aerobics students, convinced that this stuff called weight training works, approached me with their plan. "We don't want to go to a gym, we do want a group class with music and we want you to teach us how to transform our bodies into one like you have." What an exciting idea, I recall thinking. Yes, I can do that! So, in 1981, probably one of the first ever body sculpting classes began–I called it SuperShaping™. The class consisted of a total body workout using ankle weights and dumbbells in a progressive six week series.

My students immediately experienced positive changes in their bodies–changes that they had never had with aerobics alone–such as firm thighs, stronger upper body, toned arms, strength in all other activities and looser-fitting clothes! SuperShaping™ went on to be one of the first body sculpting classes featured at major corporations, taught by trained and certified SuperShaping™ instructors. It was the first step for women to experience the benefits of weight training and develop a total fitness program. As many of these women reaped the benefits of simple weight training, they expressed the desire to take it a step further–into the full-service gym. I agreed.

In l989, I returned to in-depth studies in Sports Medicine and became certified in personal fitness and strength training. I founded San Francisco's first Personal Trainer Training Course, a program to train individuals to be Personal Fitness Trainers, as well as prepare for national certification.

The Beginnings: Weight Training For Muscles & Strength

Ancient Greece is the origin of weight training. Legend has it that Milo of Crotona enjoyed a reputation of winning every battle he entered. His secret? His father gave him a baby bull. Milo loved this animal and carried it with him everywhere. As the bull began to grow, Milo continued to carry him. The bull proceeded to become heavier and Milo continued to get stronger. This was the secret that Milo had but was not even aware of–the principle of progressive resistance. To become stronger, one must continually increase the load carried or lifted.

Resistance to Resistance

So why don't most women do any resistance or weight training? The most common reason is fear of "bulking up" or appearing like Arnold Schwarzenegger. Well, I am here to tell you that we will not! The hormone called testosterone is higher in men; and that gives them the ability to develop large, bulky muscles. Women can anticipate a defined, sculpted appearance and increased strength from weight training. Women do have a certain amount of testosterone, but there just is not enough there to cause large bulky muscles. Trust me!

Muscles are the metabolic factory that burns calories. Lose them and suffer the consequences–obesity, flabbiness, loss of strength. We know the old lament that, "When I was a teenager, I could eat anything I wanted and now everything I eat ends up on my hips." Our metabolism changes and the calories were burned just by being alive (resting metabolism). Our resting metabolism decreases every year. Why? Because muscle is largely responsible for our metabolism and when we age, we lose about one-half pound of muscle per year. Therefore, our metabolism slows down. Muscle is a very active tissue that requires between thirty and fifty calories per pound per day to maintain itself. So, you can see the picture–a real concern with obesity is our gradual loss of muscle tissue.

Hooray for weight training! Obesity caused by loss of muscle is preventable and reversible at any age. Weight or strength training can add over a pound of muscle per month. More muscle means increased metabolic rate, thus putting more calories to work in our daily life. A balanced body is one that allows you to live fully. Muscular balance is the key to movement and efficiency as well as symmetry in the body.

For example, in many cases, the waistline is the area we wish to tone. This region is best addressed with a combination of cardiovascular exercise and abdominal strengthening. However, consider developing the areas above and below to change the symmetry of the waistline. Visualize this–a well developed back, chest and shoulder area enhancing your overall appearance. The toning of the hips and legs serves the same purpose–improving the appearance. Developing these areas is best accomplished with resistance training work to sculpt and change your body.

Strong. A word that women are not always, and sometimes never, described as.
Lean. An optimal description of our ideal body.
Muscular. Some, but never too much for women.

Let's clarify our ideas about muscles and strength in moving through menopause and beyond. For so long, women have turned to aerobics as the panacea for having that ideal body, but aerobics alone (AA) is not enough. You cannot increase your strength with aerobics alone. Leanness is determined by the lean muscle mass, which cannot be totally challenged with aerobics alone. Muscular in our mid-life means having tone. The ideal program to add is weight training–using weights that challenge those elusive muscles that give us the tone we need to support our changing body. In order for your body to change positively toward strength and tone you have to give it more work. We often want to stay with the same routine, then we wonder why nothing is changing. Our bodies want to stay at homeostasis (static) and will always look to adapt to your program so it can just ease into "cruise control." When you challenge your body with a new program, including more weight resistance, exercise repetitions or less rest-time between sets, it becomes more alert as it tries to figure out the new routine. Your body is trying to get familiar with the new plan–and changes result through the interaction of the brain, muscles and bones.

Can you remember when you first began any kind of exercise? Remember how quickly your body changed? It was because your magnificent assembly said, "What is this?" and quickly began re-arranging all your systems to adapt. The results–you got stronger, tighter, more flexible–everything had to adapt to the new challenge and once your body figured it out (adapted), it began to go into "cruise control" and was very happy, that you were happy, where you were, and felt no need to push or change or challenge. This very basic metabolic phenomenon is why I continually challenge my students to change their routine for maximum results. Every six weeks in my SuperShaping™ classes, I change the exercises; and each separate week brings a new challenge of more reps or a difficult method of performing the exercise, and building up to a quicker paced challenge week in the sixth week. Then, we begin all over again. My personal fitness training clients are equally challenged with new executions of exercises–by varying machines, free weights and changing order, reps and weights of exercises. You can easily do this, too, and achieve super results!

Time Spent Well

Weight training is one of the most efficient exercise systems. It is concise, and with the help of a personal fitness trainer or fitness professional, one can design a program that works the entire body in under an hour. Utilizing a fitness professional to design your program gives you the advantage of starting out right foot with sound, safe and effective exercises. Most importantly, you will learn form and alignment techniques under supervision, which will insure precise execution of exercises–probably the most important key to getting results and avoiding injuries. Just as in any sport, bad habits are hard to break. A Personal Fitness Trainer (PFT) can assure excellent performance from the beginning.

Strength Training Is Excellent Exercise for Prevention of Osteoporosis

The exciting news for women is the studies now showing the beneficial effects strength training has on bone density. The results state that strength training not only complements a weight bearing exercise program, but actually is more effective in increasing bone density. Osteoporosis (loss of bone density) concerns increase as we age. Any form of exercise that will address this is important. A full body workout addresses the entire body's bone density especially in the legs, hips, arms and spine. This may be the best reason women should adopt a strength training program as part of their workout regimen.

Flexibility vs. Weight Training

Long muscles mean flexibility. Weight training has gotten a bum rap when it comes to flexibility. You will not lose your flexibility! In fact, you may increase it somewhat if you properly train, which means that every repetition should be done as a full range of motion (ROM). Each movement should end with the movement of extending fully to beginning position. Short movements can decrease flexibility and should be avoided.

How you resist, as the muscle lengthens, is an important aspect of strength training. When we contract the muscle, it shortens. When we lengthen the muscle, if we can imagine, resisting the weight falling, you will have an important principle of safe, effective training. Using both the concentric (shortening) and lengthening (eccentric) actual contractions is key. Most weightlifters think of the shortening or contraction as the work, and then just releasing quickly, ignoring the lengthening phase as an important aspect of getting the desired results. A good rule to follow is to lift in for two counts; hold contraction two counts, and lower in four counts. This makes for a controlled, challenging, safe and effective method of lifting weights. Studies indicate slow, controlled movements decrease injury and improve muscle tone.

The Importance of Rest

Muscles need time to prepare for the next exercise session. It is as if they have to call in the reserve troops to prepare for the next battle. Whenever you lift a weight, your body has to accommodate that excess baggage by increasing the blood flow to that muscle, increasing the size of the muscle (hypertrophy), and increasing the contractile tissue. In other words, your body begins this process of preparing for you next workout immediately after you finish a session. You need to give those muscles at least forty-eight hours for this preparation process. This allows you to adapt and improve the musculature of your body. This is the reason for rest days between workouts.

Weight Training Basics? or How Much Do I Have To Lift?

The ultimate challenge–how much for the best results? Frankly, you should grunt as you overcome that last rep. Sounds strange but this is true. You should use a weight that is a challenge on the last repetition, yet you are able to execute with excellent form. You do not have to really grunt but you should be aware that you are really challenged by the last reps of each set you execute. Your PFT can assist you in form until you feel comfortable working this way.

How Do I Breathe?

Just remember TO breathe! This is a frequent question of those beginning to lift weights–when should I breathe out? The rule for breathing is to exhale on exertion or commonly at the beginning of the exercise. "Blow the weight up" is a common description that my clients find helpful. Holding the breath while straining to lift the weight is dangerous. The internal pressure increase in the chest coupled with contracted muscles can lead to limited blood flow causing feelings of lightheadedness. Most important, the increased pressure in the chest area can interfere with blood return to the heart and increase the blood pressure, a reaction known as the Valsalva Reponse. Breathing patterns will become a natural process the longer you train.

Why Weight Training?

* Slows aging process by increasing lean muscle mass which increases metabolism.
* Increases bone density; important for preventing osteoporosis.
* Adds to total, balanced fitness program.
* Efficient, concise program of 2-3, one hour workouts per week maximizes overall results.
* Decreases overuse injuries from repetitive fitness activities.
* Gives tone and sculpted appearance you cannot get from aerobics alone.
* Improves posture.
* Increases strength for "life" and in all its activities.
* Increase strength in performance of the fitness activities.
* Balances muscles groups
* Increase balance important for avoiding falling.
* Firms and tones "difficult" areas, thighs, hips, triceps, back.

"All parts of the body which have a function, if used in moderation and exercised in labors to which each is accustomed, become thereby well developed and age slowly; but if unused and left idle, they become liable to disease, defective in growth and age quickly."

HIPPOCRATES, 5 BC

CHAPTER 12

Resistance Exercises

Strength. Women. These words for many years did not go together. The psychological affect of lifting iron is quite remarkable. The thought of pushing past that point we usually want to stop. Challenging our body and mind to effort one more time. The thrill of accomplishing that last rep. All of these elements carry over to an aggressiveness that we can explore. It is okay. When circumstances arise that push past what we expected–work, family or personal–weight training with resistance exercises gives us lessons of pushing through that which we felt impossible. Choosing to put yourself under stress in weight and resistance training translates to a familiarity with unexpected stress. You will find a deep strength to meet, challenge and overcome. This is a new way of operating for us as women, but one that provides an incredible balance element to our being. We have always been strong–weight and resistance training is just the next step to power, control and masterful orchestration of life's challenges. It is the most effective fitness program to address the combination of weight gain, osteoporosis, posture concerns and life's challenge TO BE STRONG.

Life is about being strong enough to handle life. Life's activities require strength, whether its opening the bank door, carrying groceries, staying in squat position for hours as you garden, picking up children, grandchildren and great grandchildren, climbing the stairs, toting all those dresses you want to try on for that special occasion, bending to reach another copy of this book on the bottom shelf at the library for a friend, getting up from the chair, climbing those hills. Know that at any age, you can begin a program of weight training with resistance exercises that will improve your ability to function through menopause and beyond!

Real Women Do Resistance Exercises

EACH EXERCISE SHOULD BE PERFORMED SLOWLY, WITH CONTROL, CONCENTRATION AND THROUGH A FULL RANGE OF MOVEMENT. THE WEIGHT USED SHOULD ALLOW YOU TO COMPLETE NO LESS THAN EIGHT REPS AND NO MORE THAN TWELVE REPS. EXECUTION BASED ON TECHNIQUE IS SUGGESTED FOR EACH EXERCISE AS WELL AS INHALING AND EXHALING DURING EVERY REPETITION. NEUTRAL ALIGNMENT SHOULD BE OBSERVED IN ALL EXERCISES. USE TECHNIQUE INFORMATION FOR CORRECT ALIGNMENT. ALL WEIGHT TRAINING RESISTANCE EXERCISES PICTURED ADDRESS MUSCLE MASS AND BONE DENSITY. EXERCISES THAT ALSO ADDRESS POSTURE ARE INDICATED WITH (P).

SUGGESTED WARM UP: treadmill, stationary cycling, walking at low intensity for five to ten minutes. Stretch muscle groups that are focus of workout.

#1 THE LEG PRESS by Ellie

This strength exercise may be preferred if standing squats aggravate back.

Muscles: Quadriceps, gluteals.

Starting position: Seated with feet on press platform. Feet are hip width apart. Lower and upper leg form a ninety degree angle. Hands on handles and buttocks stabilized in seat.

Description: Extend legs fully to near lockout position, pause, then slowly return to starting position.

Technique: Relax shoulders and neck. Keep buttocks in contact with seat throughout exercise.

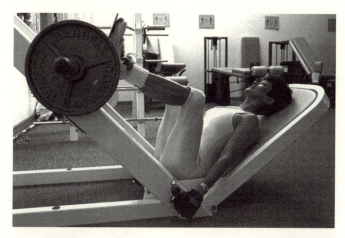

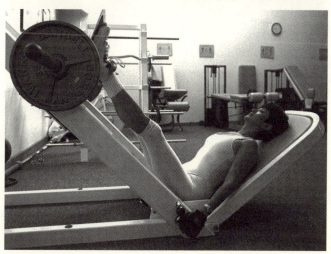

#2 THE SQUAT by Lori

Muscles: Quadriceps, gluteals.
Starting position: Stand with feet wider than hips. Bar rests on trapezius and rear deltoids with hands in wide spaced position.
Description: Lower buttocks until thighs are parallel to floor, pause and return to starting position.
Technique: Keep head up and back straight during exercise. Do not lower hips below knees.

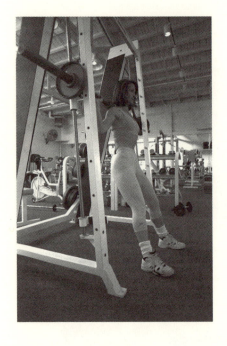

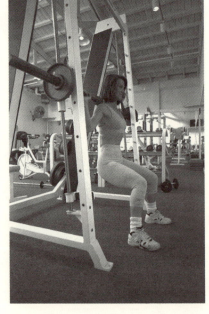

#3 THE LEG CURL by Ellie

Muscles: Hamstrings.

Starting position: Lie face down with heels hooked under roller pad. Align knee joint with axis of rotation. Place hands on handgrips. Your toes are pointed toward your knees throughout the exercise.

Description: Lift roller pad until the hamstring fully contracts, pause, and slowly lower lever to starting position.

Technique: Raise the weight so that the lower legs are at least perpendicular to the floor. Do not let hips lift more than a few inches off the bench. Do not let weight stack touch between repetitions.

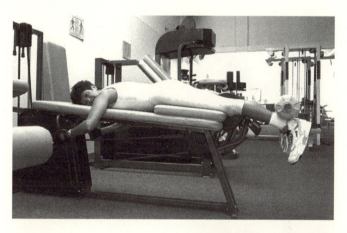

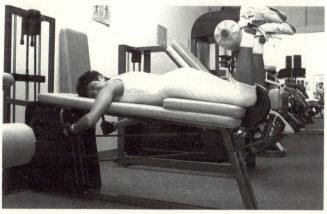

139

#4 THE LEG EXTENSION by Ellie

Muscle: Quadriceps

Starting position: Align knee joint with machine axis of rotation and place the ankles under the roller pad. Place hand on handgrips with buttocks stabilized on seat. Back is straight with eyes looking forward.

Description: Slowly lift roller pad until the quadriceps are fully contracted, pause and slowly lower to starting position.

Technique: Keep buttocks in contact with the seat throughout the exercise. Reach the extended position each rep. Use additional padding for seat accomodation for comfort and pre-stretch.

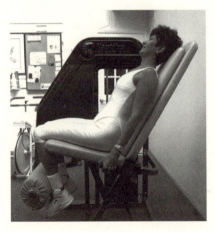

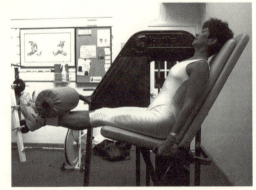

#5 THE LAT PULLDOWN by Lori

Muscles: Latissimus dorsi, biceps, rear deltoid (P)
Starting Position: Grasp the bar slightly wider than shoulders and sit with feet placed on floor, thighs secured under roller pad. Align the head and torso directly under the pully.
Description: Keeping the shoulders down, pull the bar downward to the base of the neck; pause, slowly return to starting position.
Technique: Lean forward slightly, keeping torso lifted. Stabilize the back muscles by pulling shoulder blades downward.

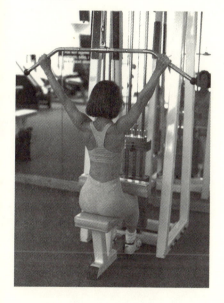

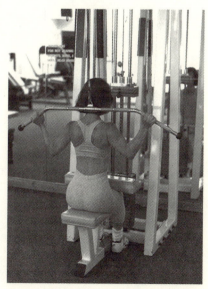

141

#6 CABLE ROWS by Lori

Muscles: Rhomboids, trapezius (P).
Starting position: Sit with feet apart and knees slightly bent. Grasp the bar with arms extended. Back is straight and eyes look forward.
Description: Pull bar to waist keeping the elbows in toward ribcage, pause, and return to starting position.
Technique: Lean slightly forward with extended arms. Do not lean back when bar is pulled to waist.

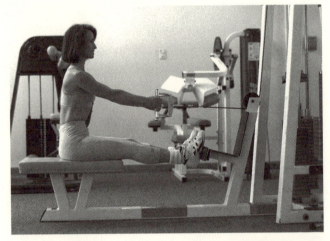

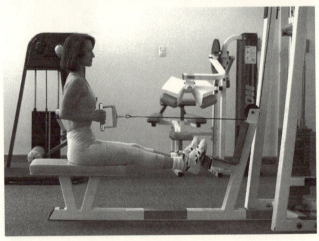

#7 THE CHEST PRESS WITH DUMBELLS by Sylviaette

Muscles: Pectoralis major, deltoids, triceps.
Starting position: Lie on bench with feet on floor or on bench. Dumbells are held in hands with arms extended above chest.
Description: Slowly lower weight to chest; pause and return to starting position.
Technique: Keep buttocks and shoulder blades in contact with bench. Keep weights parallel to floor.

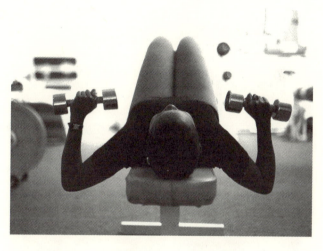

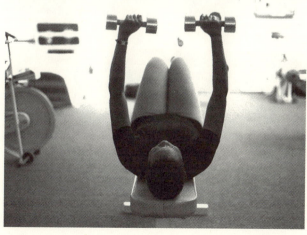

#8 THE DUMBBELL SHOULDER PRESS by Cheryl

Muscles: Deltoids, triceps.
Starting position: Stand with dumbbells at upper chest. Hands are slightly wider then the shoulders.
Description: Raise the weight so the arms extend; pause and return to starting position.
Technique: Keep back straight. Weight should extend directly over head. Do not lean backward.

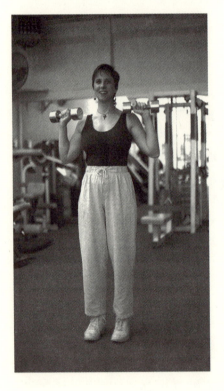

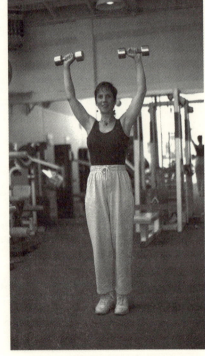

#9 THE BARBELL BICEP CURL by Lori

Muscles: Biceps

Starting position: In a standing position with arms fully extended holding barbell.

Description: Raise the barbell forward and upward completely contracting the bicep, pause and slowly return to the starting position.

Technique: Do not let your elbows come forward. Do not rest elbows on waist while lifting barbell.

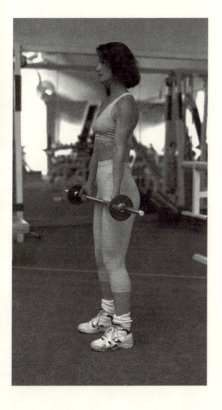

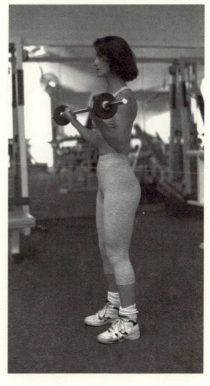

#10 THE TRICEP EXTENSION by Cheryl

Muscles: Triceps.
Starting position: In a standing position with arms bent at at elbows, grasp the tricep bar pulley.
Description: Press the pulley downward and toward your thighs, pause and slowly return to staring position.
Technique: Keep wrist straight. Keep back straight. Do not allow elbows to come forward or press into waist.

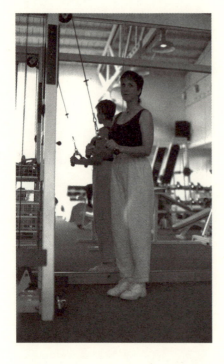

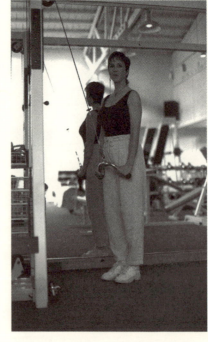

#11 THE REVERSE ABDOMINAL CRUNCH by Lori

Muscles: Rectus abdominis (P)
Starting position: Lying on back, legs extended to the ceiling, held in a position perpendicular to the floor.
Description: Contract the abdominal muscles and raise hips off the floor moving the legs upward, pause and slowly lower.
Technique: Focus on legs staying perpendicular to floor. Keep movement small and controlled. Deep upper body and head in contact with floor.

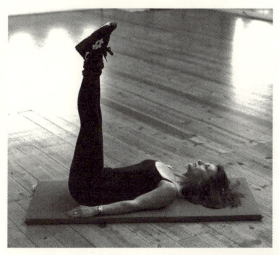

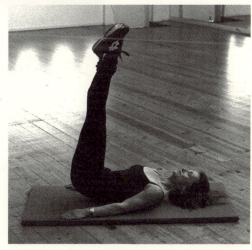

147

#12 PUSH UPS ON KNEES by Lori

Muscles used: Pectoralis major, triceps.
Starting Position: On floor with hands slightly wider than shoulders and positioned on knees.
Description: Slowly lower body until you are a few inches off the floor, pause, and return to starting position.
Technique: Do not lock arms. Maintain neutral alignment; do not drop head or sag in lower back. Control movement in lowering and pushing up.

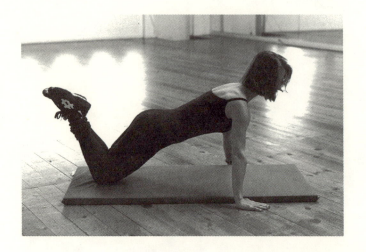

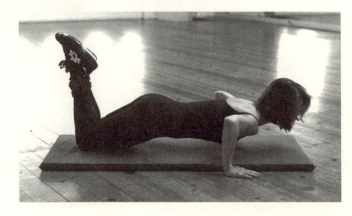

#13 STRAIGHT LEG PUSH UPS by Ellie

Muscles: Pectoralis major, triceps.
Starting position: On floor with hands slightly wider than the shoulders and legs straight.
Description: Slowly lower your body until a few inches off floor; pause and push up to starting position.
Technique: Keep neck and back in neutral position. Do not drop head or sag in lower back.

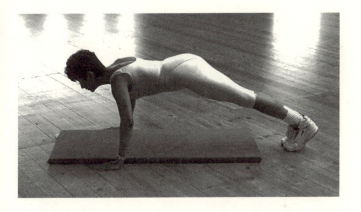

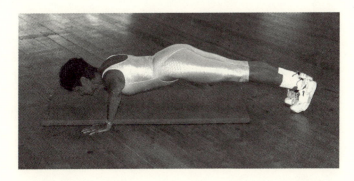

"Relax the mind and the body will follow."

ANONYMOUS

CHAPTER 13

Relaxation and Flexibility

Dateline: December 19, 1994
Happy Holidaze? at Home

Ma, you are such a scrooge!" complains my son Michael, vocally expressing my view on the Christmas season. My personal idea of a perfect Christmas vacation is lying on a beach–no tree, no gifts or any of the trimmings that go along with this holiday–unaware of the day until I overhear someone say–Merry Christmas. I just want to escape until it is all over. As the holidays approach and family and friends are gearing up, I always start thinking–how can I get out of this one? My entire family knows not to depend on me for any dinner contributions, because, somehow, I always make the great escape.

It's getting awfully close this year and I haven't planned my escape. My niece Kimberly is hosting Christmas dinner this time and has asked me to bring salad and beverages. (She is smart–give Aunt Leora items that anyone can get when she makes her inevitable escape!) Miraculously, the phone rings. "Leora, this is Pamela. I'm in Mexico at the Rancho La Puerta Spa. My roommate has canceled and I have a bed waiting for you. Get a flight down and join me."

YES! My escape route has been guaranteed for another year; compliments of a high school classmate, Pamela Price Lechtman, a professional travel writer, who just happens to be a former Editor of *Shape* magazine. My association with Pamela has given rise over the years to many series of spa trips. She would explore the decor, the food and the ambiance; while I was thrust into a major assault on fitness instructors who tried to test my true ability as I evaluated their classes.

Just in the "St. Nick" of time, an airline flight opened up and I arrived at Rancho La Puerta. Pamela and I have a wonderful time, as always, enjoying every experience this exceptional spa offers, as well as laughing into the night–paging through the 1959 Cehisean (Central High School Senior Annual) yearbook that I brought, munching a few candy bars we rationed throughout our stay.

"You have to attend Inner Journey!" Pamela exclaims as we walk to the gym at dusk. Candles are lit and placed in front of Jennifer Fox who is leading the session. It is a combination of stretch, relaxation and imagery. That powerful night, I remembered my essence, my mission in life and every event that had brought me to this moment. I remembered my first yoga class, my first meditation class, and the beginning of my life-work. Our guide Jennifer led us through an exercise where we drew a picture that was symbolic of our hopes, dreams and unresolved issues. One of my dreams was to write this book. Flying home, I felt a renewed energy. Something was about to be born. My annual great escape had brought me back to ME. You are holding my dream made reality, right now.

It is my deep belief that through flexibility exercises and relaxation practices, we can cope with the stresses we encounter during menopause and beyond. Yet this is the part of a workout that most people avoid. As soon as the instructor turns to change the mood by playing soft, relaxing music, they make the great exit. My solution to this dilemma is to stretch before and after each exercise throughout the class, which takes care of the stretching, and give a superb total relaxation at the conclusion, that, once experienced, students look forward to as the ultimate-not-to-be-missed experience.

My strengths as a teacher include: the "samurai warrior" demanding 100%-technique; communicating with clear instructions; speaking the language of the body with anatomical references to the muscles and bones; as well as the gentle voice of the yogi, soothing all the muscles that I previously challenged into relaxing submission. Most individuals spend their life uptight–not completely contracted, not completely relaxed. When you contract to the fullest, relaxation follows. This concept is the essence of the contract-relax exercises you will see demonstrated later in this chapter.

RELAXATION is when your mind's chatter ceases and tensions float away and you surrender to the "real you"–who you really are. You end these moments feeling refreshed, revitalized and filled with a crystallized energy. These moments, taken for yourself, tap your true essence, a special individual with unlimited capacity for physical, emotional and spiritual well-being; and each session reminds you of this.

When I returned from my stay with Pamela at Rancho La Puerta Spa, I was inspired to integrate my stretches throughout class, as well as my relaxation techniques and my philosophy of body-mind-spirit, and to create the class I call IN-NER STRETCH. The first class was given in January 1995 at Pacific Athletic Club and consists of total body stretches, deep relaxation using a variety of techniques and journal keeping to record year's journey of self-discovery and insights, ending with group discussion. We decided to study *Ageless Body, Timeless Mind* by Deepak Chopra. Research affirms the response from my students. Progressive muscular relaxation and imagery have been successful techniques in reducing blood pressure, neuromuscular and psychological stress.

As we are experiencing a changing body and roles during menopause and beyond, it is important to learn techniques of coping with these stresses. Choose a technique or a combination that feels right to you and practice it on a daily basis. This is not for when that moment when you go "over the edge." It is a daily practice that prepares you for that moment plus gives you relaxation and ease-of-mind. Do it every day at a set time. Shorten the length spent if you are extremely busy but do not ever skip it. Know that you will be able to complete all your tasks with a clear, refreshed and more focused mind. Incorporating these techniques in your daily life says. "I will give this time to ME first. A time that nurtures me and makes me more available to any task." Relaxation techniques take practice and patience but eventually they will be moments you look forward to.

Leora's Relaxation Exercises

Record these exercises on a cassette and guide yourself through them. Tapes of nature sounds such as rainfall and waves can be recorded in background to enhance the process. A comfortable position is important. Most techniques described are for a supine (on your back, facing up) position but can also be done seated–like at work when you need to close the door and just do it. In a supine position, some individuals experience low back discomfort when their legs are straight. Bend your knees or place a pillow under your knees or roll over to side drawing your knees up toward chest as the exercise ends if this is the case.

Deep Abdominal Breathing. Deep, slow abdominal breathing brings oxygen to all the tissues of the body and helps to relax the entire body. A regular practice of this technique, fifteen minutes twice a day, has been found effective in reducing hot flashes throughout the day. This technique is also effective at the feeling of onset of a hot flash. The act of breathing includes inhaling and exhaling. Inhalation is also referred to as inspiration. Think of inspiring the energy, feeling your desire and exhaling or expiration as ridding the body of what you do not wish. The breath is the link between your body and mind.

Technique: in a comfortable position, either seated in chair or preferably, lying on you back, eyes closed. Feel your body relax. Take in a slow, deep breath feeling your breath, filling your abdomen–expanding with the breath. Feel the breath now filling the chest, expanding the lungs as you continue to slowly inhale. Feel your breath filling your entire chest up to your clavicle (collarbone). At full inhalation, feel your entire body filled with your breath–filling your body with what you need at that moment. "I am completely relaxed." "I am calm." "I am filled with energy." Exhale slowly and deeply, from your abdomen and chest. Repeat this process for five to fifteen minutes.

Progressive Muscle Relaxation. Lying in a comfortable position with your body relaxed, begin taking in deep breaths and close your eyes. Place your arms at your side with the palms up. Bring your attention to your right leg and foot. Tighten all the muscles and hold for ten seconds and relax. Pause in relaxation for twenty seconds before going on to the next body part. Bring your attention to the following body parts in this sequence and tighten the muscles, hold for ten seconds, relax for twenty seconds: your left leg and foot, buttocks, abdomen, chest, shoulders, arms and face. As you move through your body, bring your awareness to the contracting muscle as you tense each one tighter and tighter. On relaxation, feel that body part completely relaxed. At the end, spend the time feeling a completely relaxed body. The breath is relaxed and the mind is relaxed. This exercise is very beneficial to release stress and tension.

Progressive Awareness Technique. This is similar to progressive muscle relaxation except that you will bring your focus and awareness to the body and suggest the relaxation process. In a comfortable position, take in a deep breath. Breathe in relaxation and breathe out tension. Feel your body relaxing more with each breath. Bring your attention to your right foot and leg, and feel them totally and completely relaxed. Bring your attention to the following body parts in this sequence and feel the body part to be totally and completely relaxed: left foot, leg, buttocks, abdomen, back, chest, arms, shoulders, neck and face. After going through each body part, feel your entire body totally and completely relaxed. Spend time in a totally, completely relaxed body. Remember, if you relax the body; the mind will follow.

Color Breathing. This exercise can be done standing, seated or lying in a comfortable position. Bring your awareness to your feet and legs. Breathe in the color of earth into your feet and legs. Bring your awareness to your abdomen. Breathe in the color of water in to your abdomen. Bring you awareness to your chest. Breathe in the color of air into your chest. Bring your awareness to your head. Breathe in the color of fire into your head. This is a powerful technique to balance the body. Feeling the elements of grounding in your feet and legs; flow through the stomach; deep, inspired air in the chest and the fire of creativity and energy in your head.

Hydrotherapy. Stemming from the ancient Romans, warm water has been used for centuries to soothe body and soul. It is also beneficial for a restful sleep. Water therapy is available to all of us by adding some of the natural herbal extracts found in commercial products. Kneipp®, herbal baths are my favorite. These aromatics, when added to bath water, induce a calming, soothing experience as well as relaxing tense muscles.

Sound. Music not only affects our mental state, but it can change our body's physiological response. In-depth studies indicate that a strong, regular and familiar rhythm can cause the heart to fill faster with each beat and meditative music can decrease the stress hormones, lower the blood pressure and slow the heart rate. Mellow, non-vocal music is best. Classical is ideal as well as sounds of nature: wind, waves, rainfall. See the Recommended Reading List for some of my favorites.

Flexibility

This is a very important part of your complete fitness program; and extremely important in dealing with menopause and aging. Everyone's flexibility differs, however, normal flexibility means a muscle can move through its entire length easily, the range of motion possible at a joint. Our bodies reflect stored tension, tension that comes from emotional and physical pain we have endeared our entire lives. Our bodies are the sum total of every time we have been upset, uptight, angry or hurt. To reduce stored muscular tension, it is imperative that you stretch regularly.

Why Flexibility Exercises?

A FLEXIBLE BODY REFLECTS A
FLEXIBLE MIND.

* Restore normal range of motion.
* Improve suppleness.
* Promotes efficient blood flow. Tight muscles cause pressure on capillaries, diminishing blood flow to muscles that prevents oxygen from reaching all the cells properly. Tight muscles also limit the efficiency of carrying away fatigue products that promote muscle exhaustion and soreness.
* Encourages relaxation.
* Reduces injury potential.
* Balances muscle groups.
* Improves strength, speed and endurance through the full range of motion.
* Improves coordination, agility, quickness and balance enhancing all other life activities.

Leora's Guidelines for Safe Flexibility Exercises

First, remember that static flexibility exercises are most important because they are held in a position for a specific amount of time without bouncing. Bouncing activates the stretch reflex in your muscles, causing the muscle to contract rather adapt to the stretch.

1) Always precede your flexibility workout with a warm-up that can include five to ten minutes of brisk walking, jogging, or dancing. This increases the circulation and warms the muscles; producing greater results from exercises.

2) Keep warm while stretching. Dress in warm, loose clothing. Warmth enhances the benefits of stretching.

3) Precise execution of exercise is important. Alignment and form are crucial for results. Stretch only the muscle the exercise is intended for and let the entire rest of the body relax.

4) Breathe normally with a focus on exhaling as you begin the stretch.

5) If one muscle is particularly tight, stretch the opposing muscle first. For example, if the hamstring (back of thigh) is tight, stretch the quadricep (front of thigh).

6) For balance, stretch opposing sides of the muscle.

7) Stretch to where you feel slight tension, not pain. Hold this stretch for five seconds, increasing each session to holding up to twenty to thirty seconds. If tension increases or becomes painful, ease off to a comfortable feeling.

8) Relax while stretching. Send your breath to the area and feel it warm and soften the muscle. Focus on the muscle you are stretching.

9) As your program develops and the stretches get easier, go one more step. Move deeper into the stretch in small increments until you feel slight tension again.

10) Do not compare your flexibility to another. Do not worry about how far you can stretch. Know that every time you stretch, you are improving your flexibility and overall well-being.

11) Put flexibility exercises in your life before and after each

weight training exercise. A stretched muscle contracts more efficiently and stretching carries away fatigue products, reducing muscle fatigue and soreness. Do a total body stretch with relaxation every day. Do flexibility routines before and after cardiovascular exercises like golf, tennis, or swimming.

Leora's Total Body Stretch

The following photographs illustrate a total body stretch. Isolate the stretch by feeling the stretch. You should feel the stretch where the intended exercise indicates. Alternate with the side that you stretch first. Record these stretches on a cassette with music. Enjoy!

#1 THE QUADRICEP STRETCH by Cheryl

Starting position: Lie on floor on your right side with right leg slightly bent.
Description: Bend left leg and reach back with left hand and grasp left ankle or foot. Slowly pull leg behind you until a slight stretch is felt in the thigh and front hip. Hold and breathe; slowly release. Repeat on right leg.
Technique: Hips are forward. Stretching knee is directly under the hip; not forward of the hip. Avoid arching the back.

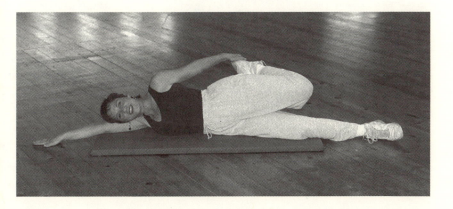

#2 THE OUTER THIGH STRETCH by Cheryl

Description: On your back, with head and torso down and arms extended to the side; bend knees and pull across the body. Slowly pull the legs toward the floor until a slight tension is felt in the hip, hold and breathe. Slowly release and repeat on other side.

Technique: Concentrate on pressing the arms and shoulders to floor, opening chest. Keep head in neutral position looking up.

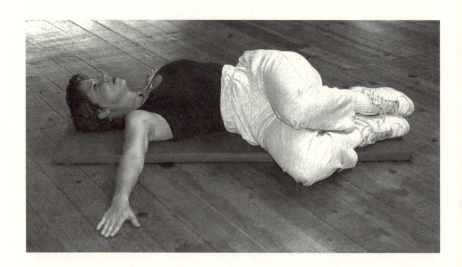

#3 THE HAMSTRING STRETCH (with bent knee) by Lori

Description: On back, with knees bent and feet on floor, extend the right leg toward ceiling. Grasp the leg below the knee. Slowly pull the leg toward you until slight tension is felt in the rear thigh. Hold the stretch and breathe. Slowly release and repeat on other side.
Technique: Keep hips on floor. Do not arch your neck.

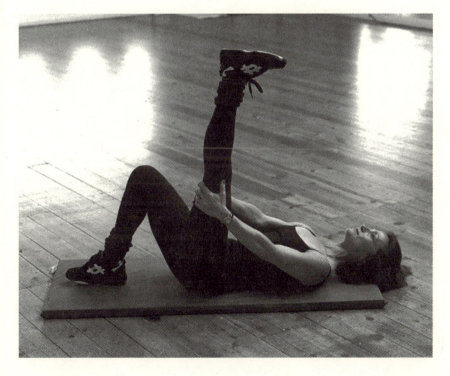

#4 HAMSTRING STRETCH (with straight leg) by Lori

Description: On back, with legs straight. Extend right leg toward ceiling keeping left leg on the floor. Grasp the right leg below the knee. Slowly pull the leg toward you until slight tension is felt in the rear thigh, from the buttocks to below the knee. Hold the stretch and breathe. Slowly release and repeat on other side.

Technique: Keep hips on the floor. Do not arch your neck.

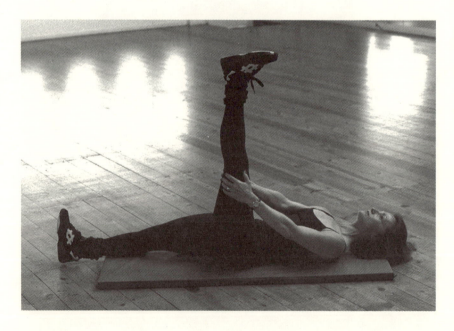

#5 INNER THIGH STRETCH by Ellie

Description: Sitting with back straight and soles of feet together, gently press knees toward floor until slight tension is felt in the inner thigh. Hold the stretch, breathe, slowly release.

Technique: Keep back erect. Press elbows down into knees for increased stretch.

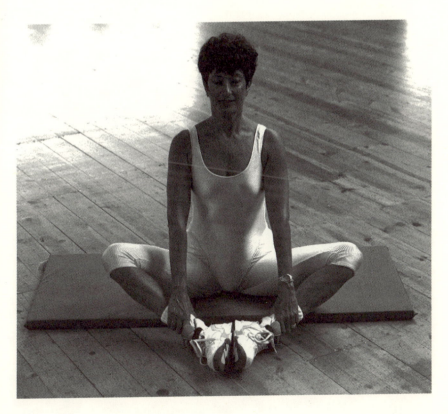

#6 TRICEPS STRETCH by Lori

Description: Seated or standing, straighten right arm toward ceiling. Bend at the elbow and touch fingertips to spine. Grasp right elbow with left hand and pull right arm toward your head until slight tension is felt in the back of the upper arm. Hold the stretch and breathe. Slowly release and repeat on other side.

Technique: Keep shoulders down and back straight. Keep head upright; looking forward.

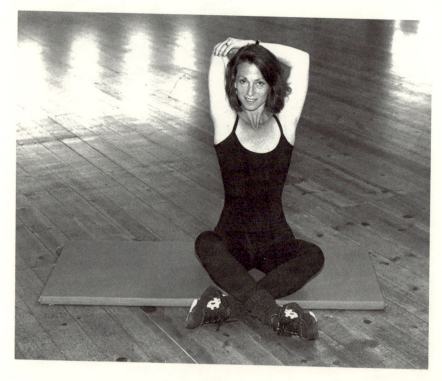

#7 LOW BACK STRETCH by Ellie

Description: On back with knees bent and arms folded under knees, gently pull knees toward chest until slight tension is felt in low back. Hold and breathe. Slowly release and relax. Repeat.
Technique: Keep face parallel to floor; do not arch neck. Lower back stays on floor.

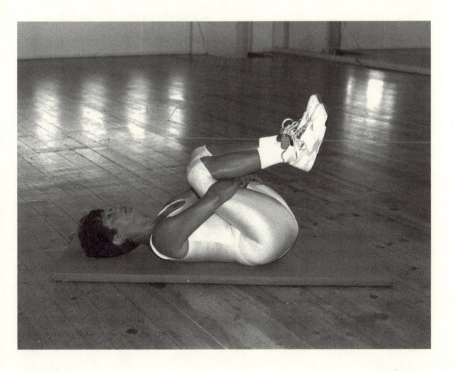

#8 SHOULDER STRETCH AND BACK EXTENSION by Lori

Description: Seated or standing, clasp hands and extend arms to ceiling until slight tension is felt in the front shoulder area. Hold the stretch and breathe. Slowly release and repeat on other side.

Technique: Keep head upright and look forward. Do not raise shoulders. Keep back upright.

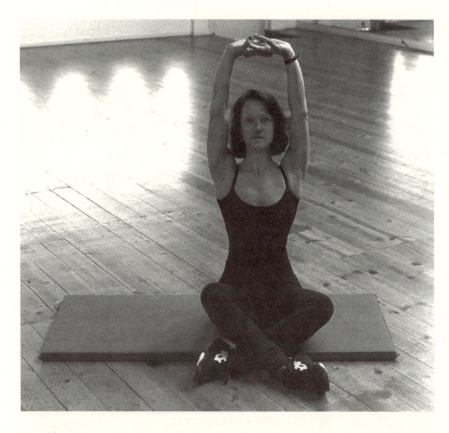

#9 THE BACK EXTENSION (STRENGTHENS THE BACK AND PROMOTES CHEST EXPANSION) by Ellie

Description:
Level I: Kneeling on the floor with knees hips' width apart and arms directly under shoulders. Feel the balance of your weight on your right leg as you lift and extend your left leg straight behind you, parallel to the floor. Extend your right arm in front of you and parallel to the floor. Hold with balance and control. Slowly bring the leg and arm down and repeat on the other side.

Technique: Eyes are focused forward, not upward. Do not arch back. Keep hips parallel to the floor. Feel strength and control in the extended arm and leg.

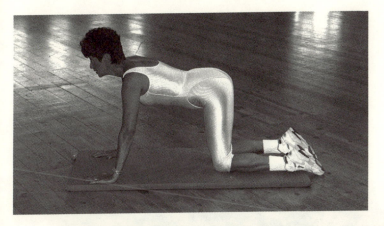

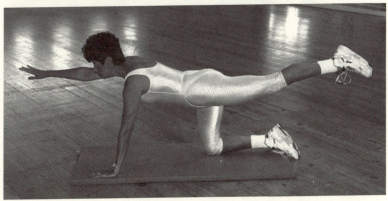

#10 BACK EXTENSION by Sylviaette

Description:
Level II: Lying down with legs straight and arms at side, slowly lift head looking forward. Slowly lift torso until rib cage is slightly off the floor. The stretch is felt in the abdomen and the contraction is felt in the lower back. Hold the position and breathe. Lower your torso and head. Relax with head turned to side and arms and legs relaxed. Repeat.
Technique: Depress shoulders as you lift. Keep neck in neutral alignment. Extend to your capability; there should not be any discomfort.

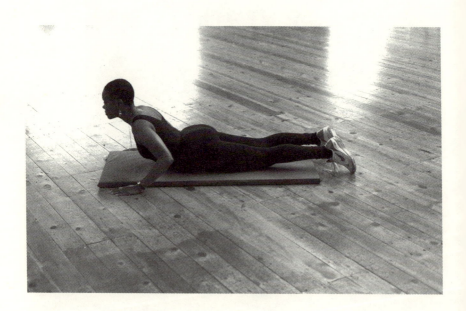

#11 THE ULTIMATE PICTURE OF RELAXATION
by Sylviaette

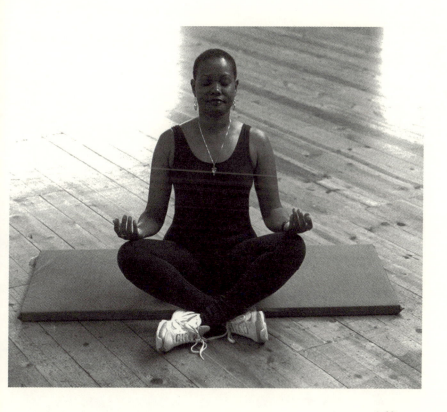

"Responding to time: where is our present knowledge rooted, if not in patterns of thought so deeply ingrained that they may be imprinted in our consciousness and genes?"

TARTHANG TULKU,
Knowledge of Freedom

CHAPTER 14

Cardiorespiratory Exercises

Dateline: Spring 1978
501 Lake Street, San Francisco
80 year young Grandmother "Rie" pays a visit

W here are they running to?", shouted Grandmother Marie (whose name I shortened to "Rie" at age 5) as she looked out our traditional San Francisco Bay window, watching the joggers pounding the pavement. Our spacious, tree lined street led to Mountain Lake Park, the Golden Gate Bridge and Baker Beach. It was a favorite route for joggers. "They're jogging," I replied. The next word out of her mouth was," Why?" I will never forget that moment. Yes, why are we out at the crack of dawn–jogging, taking an exercise class on our lunch break, lifting weights at the end of a work day, or hiking five miles on Saturday, our day "off." Because we know, deep down, that when we achieve completion of that exercise, no matter what it is, we will quite simply, FEEL BETTER AND LIVE BETTER, LONGER. Isn't that what this book is all about, anyway?

Technically speaking, the American College of Sports Medicine classifies cardiorespiratory endurance activities into three groups:

Group 1 includes physical activities in which exercise intensity is easily sustained with little variance in heart rate response: walking, aerobic dance, swimming, jogging, running, cycling, cross country skiing, stair climbing, stepping and skating. These are recommended when precise control of intensity is necessary. They can be performed in a continuous format or in an interval format. Group 1 activities expend the most energy per unit of time.

Group 2 includes physical activities in which energy expenditure is related to skill: figure and in-line skating, swimming, or highly choreographed dance exercise. These types of exercises are useful because they can be conducted in settings outside the gym–increasing mental stimulation as you learn, fostering compliance and reducing boredom.

Group 3 includes physical activities that are quite variable in intensity: soccer, basketball, racquetball, tennis, handball etc . . . Because of the variable intensity of Group 3 activities, they should include some of the base-level conditioning of Group 1. These activities tend to be group-oriented and provide greater interest for those favoring team activities along with the support of a coach.

The FIT Formula
Frequency Intensity Time

Frequency refers to the number of exercise sessions per week included in your program. To assure both cardiorespiratory fitness and maintain body-fat at near optimum level, you should exercise at least three days a week on alternate days. Increasing the frequency to five-six days a week increases the benefits but should be done gradually to avoid overuse injuries. If you are just beginning to exercise, allow at least thirty-six to forty-eight hours of rest from the activity to promote adequate recovery.

Intensity refers to the speed of exercise. Fifty to eighty percent of intensity of an exercise is recommended with the average intensity suggested between fifty to eighty-five percent.

Time refers to the number of minutes of exercise. Exclusive of the warm up and cool down, the conditioning period should last twenty to sixty minutes. The time depends on the intensity. You can exercise longer at a lower intensity. Beginners' time may include twenty to thirty minutes; compared to seasoned athlete including thirty to sixty minutes. Cardiorespiratory benefits can be obtained by splitting the time: ten minutes in morning, fifteen minutes at noon, twenty minutes in evening.

Alternative Cardiorespiratory Training Methods

Aerobic Interval Training is ideal to combat boredom and increase time of exercising. This method consists of repeated intervals of exercise interspersed with intervals of relatively light exercise. For example: stationary cycling for three minutes at a challenging workload intensity with a two minute "rest period" of cycling at low or zero resistance. How about that jogging? Try three minutes with a two minute walk in between sets.

Circuit Training is an innovative, thorough workout consisting of a series of exercise stations, with brief rest intervals between each station. Traditionally done on weight machines using low resistance and interspersed with aerobic equipment, this workout can be creatively designed in a natural setting by interspersing walking and jogging with strength, endurance and flexibility exercises.

Guidelines For Cardiorespiratory Exercises

Walking is the simplest aerobic activity, preferred because of its low injury rate, simplicity and adaptability to access, busy schedules and low, low cost.

Warm-up: walk for three to five minutes, then stretch the heel (Achilles' tendon), calf and low back.

173

Jogging/Running is slower than running and both are excellent cardiovascular exercises. Warm-up: walk-jog or jog at a slower pace then stretch the heels (Achilles' tendons), calf and hamstring, quadriceps and low back. Cool down: decrease pace and stretch same muscles.

Cycling is an excellent cardiorespiratory exercise. It is a good alternative for those having difficulty with weight bearing exercises. Outdoor: warm up–be sure to begin with relatively flat terrain in lower gears; gradually shift to higher gears and steeper terrain. Stationary bike: warm up–start with little or no resistance, then work up.

Swimming is a superior form of cardiorespiratory activity. Warm up: begin with a slow crawl and gradually increase arm stroke. Deep water aerobic classes with aid of flotation dumbbells and foot resistance are a very popular and challenging pastime for fitness. Check out water workouts at your local pool.

Stair Climbing is an effective means of attaining cardiorespiratory fitness; particularly for high-rise office workers and natives of cold climates! Warm-up: begin with fifty percent of intended speed and then work your way up.

The Next Step

There is no stopping us now! We have a wide variety of workouts available to us. Making our workout more than just the physical push, we are ready for the total body-mind-spirit connection–the connection that influences the quality of our physical results as well as mental and spiritual.

The following workouts blend the mental and physical to enhance the benefit of exercise, reduce stress and improve the overall quality of life: Pilates, Feldenkrais, wall climbing, or yoga.

❖

A special thanks to my colleague and good friend Gwen Hyatt, M.S., Exercise Science; Director of Desert Southwest Fitness, Tucson, Arizona for listening, encouraging and correcting this exercise science text. Thanks also to Randy DeLue, owner of Donnelley Square, Burlingame, for letting your beautiful studio be our photo session site.

PART FOUR

Cooling Down

"Physicians are not magicians.
They cannot look into your body.
You have to communicate to them
about what and how you are feeling!"

IRENE TEGLIA MCKAY

CHAPTER 15

Communicating With Your Physician and Health Care Team

As my seventy-two year-old client Irene so aptly put it, physicians just are not in the position to wave a magic wand. She should know, since she has survived a six-way heart by-pass, undergoes weekly kidney dialysis treatments, but has tremendous confidence in the superb team of physicians she has assembled. Why? Because Irene always communicates!

First off, let's answer a question that has been posed so many times–is menopause a medical disease? NO! It is a natural passage that all human females go through. However, certain menopausal hormonal changes are accompanied by conditions that can require medical advice and/or treatment. Here at the dawn of the twenty-first century, the method of obtaining advice and treatment is drastically changing–for the better!

We are the women who refuse to be blindly "put on" medication, or have our mood swings and hot flashes dismissed as insignificant–"all in our heads." I truly believe that we must insist on being the collaborator in the healthcare decisions we make regarding menopause and beyond. We only have this body to work with. Acknowledging, "This is my body and I am a intelligent person. I study, I read, I am here to collaborate and participate in making the best health decisions for me today and in the future," is one of most powerful assertions we can make for our healthcare. Following are my suggestions for doing just that!

Choosing the Right Type of Doctor

Although gynecologists are considered to be specialists in the health of women, many other physicians may be able to care for you. Primary care physicians, internal medicine specialists, family doctors, internists and endocrinologists all have experience in menopausal symptoms. Gynecologists have particular expertise in menopausal symptoms related to abnormalities such as bleeding, as well as prescribing appropriate hormonal therapy. Discuss your concerns and symptoms with your current physician or specialist. If you are not satisfied, interview another physician. If you develop a problem not within the scope of their expertise, insist on a referral to an outside specialist. Menopause clinics and women's health centers are now opening nationwide. Apply the same scrutiny and criteria to them that you would apply with any physician in private practice.

Beginning the Search For Doctor Right

My support group, "Mid-life & Beyond" has developed a list of physicians we trust and feel comfortable with. The method of asking friends or co-workers has proven invaluable. You may also call local hospitals to get names of doctors. Another good source is the Directory of Medical Specialists found at your local library as well as your local chapter of the American Medical Association.

Get Yourself Educated

Prepare and be well informed so that you can be the collaborator in your health care decisions. Read and study books on mid-life and menopause. (See the Appendix for my Recommended Reading List.) Attend workshops and support groups that discuss these issues. Talk with others who had similar experiences.

Make a Value Based Choice

Carefully choose your physician based on the values that you require in a medical practitioner. Check those that apply to you:
- Clinically competent to treat up-to-date woman's health needs.
- Understand female hormonal function of a woman at your age.
- Caring and compassionate.
- Willing to listen to your opinion and include you in the decision process.
- Values your time and does not keep you waiting.
- Is in group clinic setting or a solo practice?
- Are you willing to see another doctor if your preferred provider is not available?
- Do you prefer a male or female?
- Does the doctor give follow-up reports–letters, phone calls or return visits?
- Ask how doctor handles calls and emergencies after regular office hours.

Be Self-Confident

- Refuse to be intimidated by your medical practitioner.
- Communicate honestly at all times, even when you feel "uncomfortable."
- Insist on telling your "story" in your own time, in your own way.
- Declare what you expect of your relationship.

Forewarned is Forearmed

If this is your first visit to a specialist or new physician, have your medical records transferred ahead of time. Bring along any records that indicate your past and current health conditions, including:
- Screening tests results such as body fat analysis, submaximal treadmill test, mammogram, cholesterol, etc. . .
- Your present exercise and nutrition program.
- Family history indicating risk factors to heart disease, osteoporosis and breast cancer.

If the physician is perplexed with the reason you are presenting this information, you are in the wrong office!!!

Spend Valuable Time Together Wisely

- Organize your thoughts in advance. (Not while in the waiting room!)
- Make a list of your questions and concerns; write them down!
- If you are uncomfortable about a particular question, rehearse your question before the appointment. There are no stupid questions!
- If you do not understand the answer, ask for a clarification at that moment.

RECOMMENDED HEALTH SCREENING TESTS
For Women 35 Years Plus

First, it is important to understand a word frequently used in health screening tests–"baseline." It is the point or line of beginning of any act or operation. If we, the women of today, plan to collaborate in our well-being, we must have a healthcare reference point, a spring board, an initial starting ground. Participating in preventive screening tests and diagnostic testing as we mature gives us a reference point. Developing a baseline is a valuable source of information to detect any change from the beginning. These tests are our blueprints and our foundation of how our bodies are today. From our baseline, we can reflect any changes in the future. Armed with this knowledge, we can make lifestyle and health choices to positively affect those changes we notice.

Crown-to-Rump Height

Seated on a stool, you are measured from the top of your head to the bottom of your spine. This test helps assess if you experiencing more than the average loss of height that occurs with normal aging. This could be a possible sign of osteoporosis and vertebral fractures.

Frequency: every five years ages thirty-five to fifty-five, every year ages fifty-five and older.

Weight and Body Composition

Ideal weight. To calculate this, take your height in inches, multiply that figure by 4, then subtract 108. These calculations will give women of average build and weight with approximately 18-22 percent body fat. That is considered a healthy norm for body-fat of women. Obesity is defined as more than 30 percent body-fat for women.

Hydrostatic weighing is considered the "gold standard" of assessing body composition. It involves being placed underwater while seated on a chair attached to a scale. Done in sports medicine facilities.

Skin fold measurements are done with special metal calipers. Done by fitness professionals in fitness centers or sports medicine departments.

Bioelectrical impedance is based on the principle that the conductivity of electrical impulse (not enough to be painful or felt) is greater through lean tissue than through fatty tissue. Done by fitness professional.

Waist-to-hip ratio is important to indicate just where fat is accumulating on your body. Using a cloth tape measure, measure your waist at one inch above your navel. Measure your hips at the widest point. Divide waist measurement by hip measurement. Example, if your waist is 32 inches and your hip measures 36 inches, you would calculate: 32 divided by 36 =0.88. A waist-to-hip ratio greater than 0.80 may signify greater health risk. Frequency: every year.

Checks For Menopausal Status

Follicle Stimulating Hormone (FSH) Levels are the most useful test for diagnosing menopause. FSH is a hormone secreted by the pituitary gland that causes the egg in the ovary to mature. Levels above 40 indicate that you are menopausal. This test is done if you are having any menopausal symptoms and to determine hormone efficacy if you are already taking postmenopausal hormones.

Vaginal smear test takes cells from the vagina wall, in an exam similar to a Pap smear, to determine an estrogen drop causing vaginal wall to thin.

Estrogen levels are simple blood drawing and testing procedures to determine the actual amount of estrogen in the bloodstream.

Frequency: If you are experiencing any menopausal symptoms.

Check For Bone Density Loss (Osteoporosis)

If you are concerned because you are at risk for osteoporosis, or you are interested in finding out a baseline of your bone density to help make a decision about Hormone Replacement Therapy (HRT), you will want to do a bone scan. Most scans use DEXA (dual x-ray absorptionmetry). It is a non-invasive twenty minute procedure that will give you a baseline of your bone density. It costs approximately $200-300. Many insurance companies will not pay for this test, and most physicians discourage it unless you have signs of osteoporosis or conditions that preclude it. Most women I know insist on having one done at age thirty-five for a baseline even if it means paying for it themselves. The bone scan's computer program details bone loss in terms of "deviation from the norm." The World Health Organization guidelines are:

- Diagnosis of osteoporosis is two standards from the norm.
- One standard deviation below the norm, your chances of developing osteoporosis are slightly increased and having

another scan in a year is a good idea.

- If you are right at the norm, you could wait longer than a year to have another scan.

- If you have lost a higher percentage of your bone density and are two standards below normal ranges, your physician will probably recommend HRT to avoid further loss of bone density.

Blood Pressure

More than fifty percent of women over age fifty-five have high blood pressure (hypertension); defined as a reading of 140/90 or more on separate, independent readings. Normal blood pressure readings are 120/80. However, many women are unaware of their hypertension, as there is no overt symptom to suggest the disorder. Frequency: with every exam, or at least twice a year. Monthly, if on weight loss or anti-hypertensives management.

Pelvic Exam

This is a physical check for the strength of pelvic floor muscles. Your physician may insert one or two fingers into the vagina and ask you to squeeze your pelvic floor muscles. A pelvic floor assessment can be performed using biofeedback to identify and strengthen this group. Urodynamic labs and incontinence clinics are becoming more common at many of the major hospitals. Strong pelvic floor muscles help protect against urinary incontinence. Frequency: basic test, every year. Assessment test: based upon severity of incontinence.

Pap Smear

This important test will detect more than ninety percent of cancers of the cervix and nearby tissues. Since the 1940s when it was first introduced, it has reduced deaths from cervical cancer by 70%. The Pap Smear can also detect asymptomatic yeast infection, bacterial infections and can be used to determine whether the vagina is lacking in hormones. Frequency: every year.

Digital Rectal Exam
Performed in conjunction with a test for occult blood every year after 35 years.

Colon Cancer
Colon cancer is the third leading cause of death and is rather common in women over fifty. Along with digital rectal exam, you should have a stool test once a year after age fifty, as well as a sigmoidoscopy every two years after age fifty, and then every three to five years after the first two negative exams.

Breast Exam
See Chapter Four for specific guidelines and diagrams. Self: done monthly. By physician: every year.

Mammogram
One of the best ways of detecting breast cancer in the earliest stage, most curable stage is the mammogram.

A baseline mammogram is recommended between ages thirty-five and thirty-nine. Then, a mammogram every two-to-three years between ages forty and forty-nine, then every year after age fifty.

Cholesterol Screening
These tests provide a ratio of "good" cholesterol High Density Lipoproteins (HDL) and "bad" cholesterol Low Density Lipoproteins (LDL) found in your bloodstream. The recommended numbers are:

Total Cholesterol
Less than 200 mg/dl - desirable
Range of 200-239 mg/dl   -   borderline- high blood cholesterol
More than 240 mg/dl - high blood cholesterol (high risk)

HDL (High-Density Lipoproteins)
50 mg/dl or above - very good
Range of 35-50 mg/dl - good
35 mg/dl or under - increased risk factors

LDL (Low Density-Lipoproteins)
Less than 130 mg/dl - good
Range of 130-159 mg/dl - borderline
160 mg/dl and up - high risk

Triglycerides
20-140 mg/dl - normal range
140-190 mg/dl - above normal
190 mg/dl and up - high risk

The ratios of HDL to Total Cholesterol as well as HDL to LDL are as important as your overall cholesterol numbers. The American Heart Association finds that a desirable ratio of Total Cholesterol to HDL is 4:1. For example, a good range would be 200 mg/dl total cholesterol to 50 mg/dl HDL. Divide your total cholesterol by HDL to get your ratio of risk. Frequency: The baseline test between ages thirty-five and thirty-nine, every year if normal; twice or four times yearly, if you are in the borderline category, and monthly if in the abnormal range. If this is you, now is the time to consult with a physician for appropriate diet, exercise and management to be followed.
Example:
$$\frac{200mg/dl}{50} = 4.0 \text{ ratio HDL to Total Cholesterol}$$

Exercise Stress Test
If you are over fifty years of age and have high blood cholesterol or other risk factors, you should have an exercise stress test. This test is done under medical supervision and involves monitoring your heart rate and activity with an EKG while you exercise on a treadmill. This is the best way to determine your readiness to exercise and gives information to develop a fitness program suited for your needs.

Iron Status

The most common cause of iron deficiency among mid-life women is heavy menstrual bleeding, that may occur in the early years before menopause.

Tests for iron include:

Hemoglobin- the main component of red blood cells. Normal is 12-16 grams per deciliter of blood

Hematocrit- the percentage of red blood cells in whole blood. Normal is 37-47 percent.

Essentially, <u>you</u> and only <u>you</u> have the responsibility to communicate honestly with your physician and members of your healthcare team. Tell them what is going on, ask questions and be an informed collaborator in the decisions surrounding your well-being.

"Let us recognize ourselves in this old man or old woman. It must be done if we are to take upon ourselves the entirety of our human state."

Simone de Beauvoir,
The Coming of Age

CHAPTER 16

Rx for Aging . . . And Beyond

Dateline: May 16, 1995
MEMO TO: Leora
FROM: The Universe
MESSAGE: Let It Go and Get On With It
SENT: Via Experience
While Completing This Book
San Francisco, California

I believe it is important to acknowledge that there are occasional jolts to our Being that signify defiance of the process we call aging. Here is the preface to one of my most embarrassing jolts . . . I can remember, growing up back in St. Paul, Minnesota, in the early 1970s, that my mother continually "misplaced" her glasses. We were subjected to "Has anyone seen my glasses?" whenever my Mother forgot where she put them–again, practically five times a day. The usual responses ranged from Daddy, "Adelaide, why don't you have a set place where you put them?" To Brother Lyman, "Oh, not again, Ma! Why can't you remember where you last had them?" To my silent wail, "Why can't she just remember where she put her specs?" Flash forward to today and a great example of what goes around comes around. Here's me, constantly saying to my husband–"Dennis, have you seen my glasses?" And his response, "Leora, why don't you put them in a set place?" To my son Michael's one word declaration of "MOM!"

Granted, I have at least twelve fashionable pairs of glasses–in every color and shape–from tortoise rounds to serious black square rims. I am still waiting for the day I don't need them, but the Universe will not cooperate! Music tapes, magazine stand browsing material, recipes, shampoos, conditioners, tourist books, menus, bank statements, clothing labels, CD liner notes, letters, directions on every thing–manufacturers just don't get it! I need large print because I can't read the type and I refuse to wear glasses! I am now imitating my Mother's squinting technique and I said I would never do that!

Unsolicited advice has always poured in: "You can get one contact lens for close reading, Leora. It takes a helluva long time to get used to . . . but it works." "Why don't you just wear your own glasses, Leora." "You look good in glasses, Leora. What's the big deal? Bifocals are improved . . .you can't see the line."

The bottom line that I do not want to see is:
Loss of Vision = Aging
I HATE THIS PART OF AGING! I CAN TAKE MOST OF IT! BUT LOSING MY EYESIGHT–THIS I HATE! IT'S A HASSLE TO ALWAYS HAVE TO HAVE THESE DAMN GLASSES ON TO READ ANYTHING.

So, here I am, in the middle of May, forging ahead in life, and suddenly, at 2:30p.m., I had a tremendous urge to indulge in a meal-from-hell. I'm not sure what triggered it, but the urge wasn't going away, so I placed the order: chicken fried steak with mashed potatoes and gravy. I sat and devoured this sin meal. (Please note this is not a frequent habit of mine, but an urge that has to be met immediately in order for me to keep my sanity!) My morning hours had been spent training clients and my afternoon included two more training sessions as well as teaching a SuperShaping™ class.

At 3:30p.m., I went to the Telegraph Hill Athletic Club and prepared for my sessions. A righteous tooth brushing felt like a good thing to wash the sin meal from my mouth and conscience, along with an Ibuprofen tablet for a hip injury that I had sustained several weeks before. I placed the Ibuprofen down on the sink, enjoyed my vigorous tooth brushing, then took the tablet. It felt a little rough going down, so I swallowed another glass of water. I went to put the cap on my toothpaste and it was nowhere to be found. Instead, I found the tablet–OH MY GOD, I SWALLOWED THE TOOTHPASTE CAP!

My first thought was–Leora, how stupid can you be?–quickly followed by–Oh, it will be okay. I went on to finish my hectic day, after eating a bagel and flushing down plenty of water. At 8:00p.m., I went back to my studio and recorded some music, all the while trying to ignore the fact that I had a toothpaste cap in my body. I really did not have any acute discomfort, just an awareness of the "invader" mid-chest. Around 9:30p.m., I came home and told my husband Dennis about my stupid deed. He inquired right then and there, "Do you want to go to the hospital?"

"No, I will be fine," I said, even though I am thinking–I hope this cap inside me is not a big thing. As I sat down to write around 11:40p.m., all my nursing education and training began to paint vivid pictures of all the possibilities surrounding this increasing pain in the middle of my chest--a perforated esophagus or an obstructed stomach? I awaken Dennis to the plan that he had suggested hours ago by finally announcing, "I have to go to the hospital!"

May 16, 4:00a.m. Dennis and I drag up the house steps and fall into bed after our trip to the emergency room, which eventually produced an x-ray that indicated the "cap invader" was on its way down and I would be just fine. At 10:00a.m., I placed a call to my optometrist. Yes, this is Leora Myers. I would like to make an appointment for an examination for eye glasses and contact lenses.

So now you can see the real Leora--indulging in "sin" foods from time-to-time and having undeniable issues with some aspects of aging. However, the tale I've described is not to be taken too lightly. I could have ended up in the emergency room for something far more serious, simply for failing to use my eye glasses.

Another jolt of discovery to come out of this experience was realizing how the relationship I share with my husband has evolved over the years and most importantly, how concerned he really is about my welfare. Not once did he complain about getting out of bed at 11:40p.m., even though he had suggested going to the hospital earlier–no "I told you so's" or "I've told you to wear your glasses!" Relationships unfold as we age. What once would have been a shortness in temperament had changed to a pause of concern and caring for the well-being of a life-mate.

Aging

The study of aging is just beginning to be an active, scientific investigation. Initial research does indicate that what were once considered normal processes of aging are really results of inactivity and lifestyle choices. No kidding! Hooray, the essence of this book is choosing fitness and lifestyle choices for well-being, longevity and quality of life. Many of the changes we attribute to old age are actually an accumulation of bad habits (except for poor eyesight)! We can slow down the aging process. We do have control over many physical changes. So, here is more information–some R_x (prescriptions, if you will) to help you create a new vision of aging without poor eyesight, skin and hair loss–some practical knowledge and strategy for maximizing the prime of your life.

Eyes

Myopia or nearsightedness is most common problem of aging eyes of those under age forty-five. Presbyopia or farsightedness is most common concern of aging eyes over forty years old. Corrective lenses either in glasses or contacts can easily correct these conditions. (Yes, I now wear my own glasses every day!)

- Never look directly into sun.
- Wear ultraviolet absorbing lenses in sunglasses or eyeshades.
- When doing close work at a computer, take frequent breaks, at least every two-to-three hours, closing your eyes and focusing on faraway object. Use sufficient lighting always.
- Chronic alcoholism is related to dimness of vision. Research suggests that chronic alcohol abuse is usually accompanied by poor nutrition which may be the real cause.
- Balanced nutrition is critical. Maintaining a diet rich in Vitamin A, C, E, Folic Acid and Zinc is important.
- Avoid mega-dosing vitamins to make up for lost time and nutrients and focus on a diet that is rich in fresh, unprocessed food.

Skin

As the body's largest organ, the skin protects us from the harsh elements, holds everything together, while remembering every smile, grimace and laugh. Our skin is the part of the body with which we face the world and the announcer of aging–how we served the sun, how we react to happy and sad times and what our parents gave us as "line heritage." For many years, I have blamed my father for the two creases between my eye brows. Recently, I found a picture of my first boyfriend and me. There we were, standing in front of Great Grandmother Georgianna's house in our romper suits. I was two years old and had a scowl on my face that was proof positive that I have been creasing my brow just that way for a lifetime!

FITNESS OPTIONS

-Regular exercise nourishes the skin by increasing blood flow, eliminating waste through sweating, and promoting collagen production. (Visit Part Three of this book for specifics!)

LIFESTYLE OPTIONS

- Avoid sun and excessive tanning since this leads to premature wrinkling.
- Use sunblock on a regular basis with a Sun Protection Factor (SPF) of at least fifteen.
- If you are in the sun, avoid tanning between 10:00a.m. and 2:00p.m. Standard time, when ultraviolet rays are the strongest.
- Rapid weight loss causes skin to wrinkle. Slow, gradual and steady weight loss allows skin to adjust to change and lessens the wrinkling effect.
- Drink six to eight glasses of water a day. This will help to maintain hydration of the collagen in the skin.
- Keep skin moist. Low humidity, dry climate and windy conditions make skin prone to wrinkles. Moisturizers prevent water loss from skin.
- Do not smoke; for many reasons, but think of this skin-related trauma–smoke rises up to face, dries the skin and causes lines around mouth leading to premature wrinkling.
- Have a balanced nutrition plan including nutrients for the skin like foods rich in Vitamins A, B, C and Riboflavin. Consult with your dietitian regarding appropriate dosages.
- Decrease alcohol intake to avoid premature wrinkling.

The Hair

Hair is probably the loudest bearer of the message that you are aging. When does this happen? You see that first hair under your chin; the hair on your head begins to thin; your pubic hair begins to decrease; the gray hair in your scalp rises. Did you know that you lose an average of 50-120 hairs per day? Thus, about 30,000 hairs per year are replaced by new ones. As we age, the replacement process just becomes a bit slower, lighter or faded. Hair changes tend to begin in the early forties, but much of the damage stems from abuse and carelessness before age forty. You can combat these changes without necessarily increasing your trips to the beauty salon.

Lifestyle

- Ultraviolet sun rays are damaging to the hair, causing the shaft to dry and ends to split. Cover your hair when in the sun and use moisturizing conditioners in hot, dry climates.
- Most colorings, chemical treatments, permanent waves and straighteners will cause damage. Follow each treatment with a product that conditions and protects hair shaft.
- Excessive brushing and/or too vigorous stroking can cause hair loss. Brushing wet hair is more damaging. Use your fingers to de-tangle.
- Poor nutrition and diets low in protein, iron, B vitamins and essential minerals can cause hair damage and loss. Overdosing on Vitamin A can cause baldness. Consult with your dietitian regarding dosages. (The good news is that true female baldness is a rare prob lem and usually has a genetic basis.)
- Stress can cause hair follicles to go into a resting stage and then shed.
- Blow dryers, with their raging hot air can cause hair to become parched, brittle and split. Use a low temperature and do not use one every day.
- Excessive and unwanted hair can be caused by the drop in women's estrogen levels due to menopause. Drugs to lower male hormones in the body can be used but may have side effects. Tweezing, waxing or using

depilatories help. Permanent removal can be done
by electrolysis. Consult a licensed professional.
- Gray hair is caused by a natural decrease in pigment as we
age. Is this gray premature? Caused by stress? Caused
by vitamin deficiency? Whatever the true answer,
here are some suggestions: stay natural, have highlights professionally done or use permanent color.

. . . And Beyond

Life expectancy in 1900 was forty-seven years. Today, it is
ranging from seventy-eight to eighty years, putting "mid-
life" at around forty. Is "old" an age, an attitude, a way of
living? What is your definition?

Aging is a transition into another phase of life. We have had
a long history of transitions–going through them and sur-
viving. They have never been a piece of cake, yet we have
survived and derived the strength and wisdom to challenge
the next one. Because we tend to forget, I would like to jog
your memory.

First Transition: Birth. Here we are floating in warm fluid,
all our needs are taken care of, and suddenly one day, the
rumble begins and we make our first major transition–begin
pushed down a tight, narrow canal, forced out of our warm
habitat into a cold, noisy, bright world. Here, you have to
breathe on your own, suffer through wet diapers until you
are changed, and cry intensely for food and attention. In
this transition into infancy, our trust is developed and grows
and is nurtured, by those who care for us.

Second Transition: Early Childhood. We now find out that
it is up to us to get what we want. So we begin to act more
independently. Walking, expressing our viewpoint as we
begin to be self-reliant, and displaying our willpower. We
get a little pushy!

Third Transition: Pre-School. Time to go for it! Our confidence grows because we are uninhibited by fear and forget
failures easily. We now are figuring out the benefits of sharing and being cooperative.

Fourth Transition: School Age. Time to show our competency. A Time to forget all those dreams, get down to some serious stuff. We now learn the lesson that in order to produce, you have to apply yourself as well as develop certain skills. No fooling around now, this is serious business.

Fifth Transition: Adolescence. Childhood is O-V-E-R. Physical growth and sexual maturation kick in along with fluctuating hormones and our moods. We seek our true identity and we are greatly influenced by how others view us. Peer acceptance and career goals are important issues and answering the question–WHO AM I? dominates.

Sixth Transition: Adulthood. We now have a sense of identity and seek relationships of mutual trust, respect and intimacy. It is important that we do not lose our individuality to the relationship. We need to share and extend our identity.

Seventh Transition: Mid-life. Where we evaluate our life to date and look at our sense of purpose. We thoroughly examine our identity, life event and contemplate our future.

As we are living longer we are able to experience mid-life. And mid-life is another transition. Mid-life is a developmental stage that has not been studied because of human's short life span in the past. I have come to view this as a Developmental Transition, a phase of life that can be positive, productive, healthy. A stepping stone for the next phase in our cycle of life instead of a time of deterioration and decline. Doesn't it resemble another stage of development we experienced? Adolescence: the hormones, new roles, new lifestyle, peer acceptance and career goals. It involves letting go of a particular self-image and beginning anew.

If you will notice, every transition begins with an ending. MENOPAUSE is the end of the menstrual cycle and the connection for many of us to being a woman–the capacity to bear fruit. Beyond menopause, the fruit we bear is of personal transformation. We are no longer confined. We are able to express our very unique spirit with a wisdom to tackle the challenges of today and tomorrow–the challenges that really are gifts to show us our infinite abilities. Old dreams become new realities and quests to be conquered with today's self-image. Does this give you a clue about why many people become successful in later years? Ghandi discovered his real mission of non-violent resistance at age fifty. Look at the successes of Grandma Moses and Colonel Sanders!

We have been busy doing the day-to-day worldly business and now we are free to do our true work of self-realization. Women have lived too long not to reap the benefits of this time in our lives. We have too much depth of experience, judgment and wisdom to slide into decline. I am proud to say that no, I am no spring chicken! I am a Phoenix with a "not born yesterday" wisdom!

I want to leave you with just a few words of wisdom for tackling the "Beyond" part of the Big M. Please . . . read and mentally discuss all the physical, emotional and spiritual issues before you at this time of transition. Make choices and act on improving your quality of life. Find medical professionals you trust. Know that you are capable of choosing fitness and wellness. Join with other pioneering women committed to creating a new vision of aging. Be filled with the positive, productive mastery of life that only the blessings of fitness of body, mind and spirit can bring.

The spirit in me salutes the spirit in you!

Make The World Your Gym

No equipment required!

- Climb steps instead of using elevators or escalators.
- Leave the car and walk.
- Walk the mall, the dog, and do it with a loved one.
- Do Kegel exercises wherever you are.
- Coordinate a walk and shop club.
- Park farther away from restaurants and stores.
- Take a hike.
- Skip stones in the stream.
- Smell the roses.

APPENDIX

YOUR FITNESS PLAN FOR LIFE

Now is the best time in your life to answer these questions. This is your personal plan for optimal well-being throughout your life. You will not be graded on what you write. The sky is the limit. Choose a special journal or workbook to record the following information. Arrange a quiet place and time for this exercise.

Using the information, ideas and inspiration in this book, write in detail:
What are your personal criteria for how you wish to live the rest of your life?
What are your personal criteria for optimal well-being for the rest of your life?
Seeing each part as a chapter in your journal, describe your life involvement at each age:
1. Physical Fitness
2. Nutrition
3. Exercise Program
4. Relationships
5. Career
6. Family
7. Intellectual Pursuits
8. Spiritual Attitude.
Add any components important to you.

(continued next page)

AGE

40_____

50_____

60_____

70_____

80_____

90_____

100_____

110_____
complete to your age expectancy.

Review this journal regularly and add information on your immediate goals. Feel free to edit, delete and embellish as your life dictates.

PLAN THE REST OF YOUR LIFE!

RECOMMENDED READING LIST

These resources are arranged under topic headings to assist you in discovering more specific information about key *Menopause & Beyond* topics. Happy reading!

MENOPAUSE: GENERAL READING

Menopause Naturally by Sadja Greenwood, M.D. (Volcano Press, Volcano, California, 1992, Updated Version)
This is an excellent primer on menopause. It is easy to read and gives both sides of the hormone controversy. Dr. Greenwood is my inspiration and the person who told me to write my own book.

Making Sense of Menopause by Faye Kitchener Cone. (A Fireside Book, Simon & Schuster, New York, 1993)
Interviews with over 150 women give a personal touch to this well-researched book. An added plus: special section for you to copy and give to the man in your life.

Stay Cool through Menopause: Answers to Your Most Asked Questions by Melvin Frisch, M.D. (The Body Press/Perigee, New York, 1993)
This book gives an easy-to-understand, comprehensive consultation with a physician about all the aspects of menopause. Excellent reference for questions.

Natural Menopause: The Complete Guide to a Woman's Most Misunderstood Passage by Susan Perry and Katherine A. O'Hanlan, M.D. (Addison-Wesley Publishing Company, New York, 1992)
Although this entire book is excellent, its strength lies in its ability to clearly illustrate the decision about HRT based on the research and the consciousness of individual choice.

The Menopause Self-Help Book by Susan Lark, M.D. (Celestial Arts, Berkeley, California, 1990)
This book focuses on alternative approaches to menopause including vitamins, herbs and specific remedies for individual problems.

EMOTIONAL & SPIRITUAL

Woman at the Edge of Two Worlds by Lynn V. Andrews (HarperCollins Publishers Inc., New York, 1993)
This is a wonderful book that gave me great inspiration and hope. It is about menopause, spirituality and how menopause is the gateway into women's most sacred time. She details with stories about the significance of menopause.

The Four Fold Way: Walking the Path of the Warrior, Teach, Healer and Visionary by Angeles Arrien, Ph.D. (HarperCollins West, San Francisco, 1993)
This book illustrates the wisdom of ancient teachers showing us how to balance our lives.

Inner Athlete: Realizing Your Fullest Potential by Dan Millman (Stillpoint Publishing, PO Box 640, Walpole, New Hampshire, 1994)
Dan illustrates how to rediscover your full potential as a "natural athlete" and apply those principles to transforming training into daily personal growth and discovery.

Meditations: Creative Visualization and Meditation Exercises to Enrich Your Life by Shakti Gawain (New World Library, San Rafael California, 1991)
This book contains Shakti Gawain's most popular meditations and visualization techniques.

SEX

The Magic of Sex: The Book That Really Tells Men About Women and Women About Men by Mariam Stoppard, M.D. (Dorling Kindersley, Inc., New York, 1991)
The title really says it all!

Men Are From Mars, Women Are From Venus: A Practical Guide for Improving Communications and Getting What You Want in Your Relationships by John Gray, Ph.D. (HarperCollins, New York, 1992)
Should be required reading for every woman as well as her partner! Highlights are also available on a sixty minute audio tape. Superb!

NUTRITION

Dr. Dean Ornish's Program for Reversing Heart Disease by Dean Ornish, M.D. (Ballantine Books, New York, 1990)
Excellent guide for those serious about taking the necessary steps to long term health and well-being.

Super Nutrition For Menopause by Ann Louise Gittleman (Simon & Schuster, New York, 1993)
A very good guidebook in the realm of nourishment.

EXERCISING

Any book by Kenneth H. Cooper, M.D., MPH
This man is recognized as inventing the word aerobics. All of his books and materials have my highest recommendation. They are easy to read and give knowledgeable explanations of physical fitness.

Stretching by Robert Anderson (Self-published, Robert Anderson, Post Office Box 767, Palmer Lake, Colorado 80133, 1992)
Easy to understand everyday stretches as well as sport-specific stretches.

AND BEYOND (TRENDS)

Age Wave: The Challenges and Opportunities of An Aging America by Ken Dychtwald, Ph.D. (Jeremy Tarcher, Inc., Los Angeles, 1989)

I regard Ken as one of my life mentors. With diligence and heart, he illustrates in technicolor the most important trend of our time–a positive and hopeful new vision of aging.

The Popcorn Report by Faith Popcorn (HarperCollins, New York, 1991)

Detailing trends, this book reveals how to chart the future's impact on your work, home and life. Suggested reading for those planning to be around in the year 2000.

Ageless Body, Timeless Mind by Deepak Chopra (Crown, New York, 1993)

It's possible! The title says it all!

MUSIC

Steve Halpern, the New Age music pioneer and visionary. All his music is wonderful. For a catalog, call 1-800-909-0707 or write: Sound Rx, 524 San Anselmo Avenue, Suite 700, San Anselmo, California, 94960-2614

Paul Horn. *Inside the Great Pyramid* (Mushroom Records, 1977)

Flesh Bones. *Skeleton Woman* (Silver Wave Records, 1993)

Suzanne Chiana. *Private Music* (Private Music, 1994)

ORDERING INFORMATION

Leora Myers Fitness Programs
Leora Myers, RN
333 Garces Drive
San Francisco, CA 94132

_____ I am interested in learning more about Leora Myers' programs!

_____ Speaking to my organization_____ on _____

_____ Mid-life and Menopause Workshops

_____ *Midlife & Beyond®* Support Group

_____ Sound Fitness®, Leora Myers' Personal Training Audio Tapes

_____ Please call me right away! The best time to contact me is:_____

_____ Please place my name on your mailing list for future information.

You can order additional copies of this book by using this form.

Please Send _____copies of *Menopause & Beyond: A Fitness Plan For Life* at $12.95 each plus shipping and handling @ $2.00 per edition. (CA residents only, add 7.75% Sales Tax) to:

NAME_____

STREET ADDRESS

_____

CITY_____STATE_____ZIP_____

TELEPHONE

DAY_____EVENING_____

My personal check or money order is enclosed, made payable to Leora Myers.

Quantity discounts are readily available. Please inquire! Thanks for your interest in your health and fitness!